BODYMIND ENERGETICS

BODYMIND ENERGETICS

Toward a Dynamic Model of Health

MARK SEEM, Ph.D.

with Joan Kaplan

HEALING ARTS PRESS
ROCHESTER, VERMONT

Healing Arts Press
One Park Street
Rochester, Vermont 05767

Text illustrations by William P. Hamilton.

LIBRARY OF CONGRESS CATALOGING-IN-PUBLICATION DATA
Seem, Mark.
Bodymind energetics : toward a dynamic model of health / Mark Seem
with Joan Kaplan.
p.   cm.
Reprint. Originally published: Rochester, Vt. : Thorsons
Publishers, c1987
Includes bibliographical references.
ISBN 0-89281-246-X
1. Acupuncture—Philosophy. 2. Mind and body. 3. Typology
(Psychology) 4. Personality—Physiological aspects. I. Kaplan,
Joan. II. Title.
[RM184.S37 1990]
615.8′92—dc20   89-49072
                                                                CIP

Text design by Leslie Phillips.

Printed and bound in the United States

10 9 8 7 6 5 4 3 2

Healing Arts Press is a division of Inner Traditions International, Ltd.

Distributed to the book trade in Canada by Book Center, Inc., Montreal, Quebec

Distributed to the health food trade in Canada by Alive Books,
Toronto and Vancouver

To the memory of Michel Foucault, whose Nietzschean perspective and guidance set me on the Way; Olga Bernal, whose early support encouraged me to remain an engaged thinker; Lourdes Alvarez-Klein, whose influence is present throughout this discussion; and to my children, Illyan and Anya Kaplan-Seem, who taught me to perceive phenomenologically.

M. D. S.

Contents

Author's Acknowledgments

Many friends and colleagues have given me invaluable help in clarifying and articulating the ideas presented here, none more so than Lourdes Alvarez-Klein, a Mexican physician, acupuncturist, and homeopath who introduced me to the work of Georg Groddeck and spent numerous hours commenting on the text. Her insights and clinical perspective prodded me to transform my way of working with patients as well as my thinking about health and illness.

Robert Duggan, an acupuncturist, president of the Traditional Acupuncture Institute, and a leader in the development of American acupuncture, made many crucial comments on the manuscript and generously extended his support and encouragement. I would like to thank Philip Kaplan, whose logical thinking led me to clarify many formerly obscure passages; Jeannette Kossuth, for her helpful suggestions concerning the format and structure of the text; Dr. Gerald Epstein, who encouraged me along the way; and Jan Resnick, who made valuable professional observations. I would also like to thank Eric Stephens, Harris Dienstfrey, Dr. Leon Hammer, and Robert Dunn, for helpful comments on early versions of the manuscript.

Thanks to Ehud Sperling, president of Thorsons, for taking on this project in its earliest stages and for stimulating me to be forceful in its presentation, and to Leslie Colket, my editor at Thorsons, whose valuable comments and editorial questions resulted in greater clarity at many points in the text.

Finally and foremost, I would like to thank Joan Kaplan, my wife, who never tired of listening to these ideas in all phases of their development over the past five years, and who took on the tremendous task of turning a somewhat wild manuscript into a more manageable, generally more agreeable presentation. While I must assume all responsibility for the ideas presented in the following pages, this book would have proved difficult going for many readers had it not been for her careful rereading and reworking. Whenever the reader encounters the pronoun *I*, it refers to the author, and *We* refers either to the general community of American acupuncturists, or to those cited here, depending on the context, who see the coming of a new bodymind paradigm.

When the reader encounters a particularly pleasing passage, this is undoubtedly due to the talents of Joan Kaplan, whose linguistic abilities far outweigh my own.

Mark D. Seem
Fire Island, New York
July, 1986

Co-Author's Note

Mark Seem and I share a home, children, and a philosophy of life. Our talents, however, are not equally distributed.

The force behind this book belongs to Mark. The knowledge, the ideas, and the vision it is built on, as well as the clinical practice that is its foundation, are his.

For my part, I have had the pleasure of taking an already fascinating manuscript and helping rework it by asking hard questions, demanding comprehensible and interesting answers, and in some cases rewriting passages to make them say, in a more organized and articulate fashion, what Mark intended them to say.

Joan Kaplan

Foreword

In real life a person is both an embodied mind and a mindful body. It seems, therefore, that the concepts of 'mind' and 'body' as separate entities are abstractions from the wholeness of human beings as they actually exist. Yet, clearly, there is also a distinction to be made between the two. Such abstractions are as real, pertinent, and necessary as a person having a name, a biography, or a foot.

No medical theory or practice has had an easy time with this dichotomy. No simple, ready-made answers to the interaction between mind and body await us in remote China, India, or Egypt; in nineteenth century Germany or twentieth century Vienna or Chicago. Even medical systems that supposedly have less difficulty with the dilemma have had to contend with it. For example, chapter twenty-four of the oldest Chinese medical textbook, the *Yellow Emperor's Canon of Internal Medicine* (200 BC) has a famous discussion of how to treat a person whose bodily and psychospiritual symptoms are incongruent and have divergent indications. In the course of its development, Chinese medicine elaborated various perspectives on bodymind interaction. But Cartesian philosophy in the West and, later, modern technological biomedicine have actually rendered the differentiation between body and mind dysfunctional, seriously impairing the ability of scientific doctors to provide adequate health care. The rise of modern psychology and psychiatry is partly a response to this problem.

In *Bodymind Energetics*, Mark Seem has undertaken a unique dialogue between two medical systems that rarely communicate. His remarkable and innovative work explores new possibilities, using acupuncture to inform modern psychology and modern psychosomatics to expand contemporary acupuncture practices. This book does not repeat the supposed "eternal truths" of any one system. Rather it engages, explores, criticizes, reflects, observes, and wonders from its own authentic point of departure.

While readers may not agree with all of Dr. Seem's observations and interpretations, they cannot help but be informed and encouraged to consider anew the potentials that need exploring in their own theoretical and clinical work. *Bodymind Energetics* is a brave and courageous exploration of an ancient dilemma from an entirely new perspective, providing valuable insight to acupuncturists, psychologists, medical doctors, and all health care providers and their patients. This dialogue will not only enrich the two participant medical systems but will also contribute to the entire field of health, medicine, and healing.

Ted Kaptchuk
Author of *The Web That Has No Weaver*

I

BODYMIND ENERGETICS

1

A New Paradigm of Health and Bodymind Energetics

Healing is not just a property of the physical body . . . we are all mind-bodies, so that healing, like health and illness, must also be psychosomatic.[1]

Andrew Weil

HEALING THE BODY/MIND SPLIT

The issue of the relationship between mind and body is as old as Western civilization itself. Through a complicated history of exclusions and omissions, the current medical model operates as if there were a split between the psyche and the body process, where the body constitutes the only legitimate arena for medical intervention and the mind remains the exclusive domain for psychological inquiry. Such a position denies the spirit or soul of the individual seeking treatment, while it ignores the fundamental connection between the bodymind and the forces of the outside world.

Any serious attempt to move beyond the modern medical model, in order to develop a new paradigm of health care focused on the maintenance of general well-being and the prevention of illness, must begin with healing this body/mind split, particularly in the thinking of health care professionals themselves, and in the conception of health held by the general public. A basic aim of this book is to articulate the philosophical position that underlies this split and has resulted in the separation of the academic disciplines of mind and body. With

3

this clarification, we shall be in a better position to explore new ways in which body and mind therapies might be integrated.

In the following pages one such integration, that of acupuncture energetics and psychosomatics, will be explored.

The Western body/mind split dates back at least as far as the Judeo-Christian ascetic ideal, wherein the soul was viewed as prisoner of the body. The goal of an ascetic life was to rise above the body, through sacrifice and self-discipline, and the spiritual quest thus conceived was a disembodied phenomenon.[2]

In 19th century Germany, where a critique of the Judeo-Christian ascetic ideal was being formulated, Freud was working to gain recognition for the importance of the psychic drives and their vicissitudes,[3] while other thinkers, such as Nietzsche, were postulating the need to develop a new morality free of this Judeo-Christian asceticism.

Working for a *retrieval of the human body*,[4] Nietzsche sought to reevaluate the morality of his time and to move beyond the split between body and spirit by spiritualizing the body itself. He created a philosophy of forces (the Will to Power, the Eternal Return, *ressentiment*) that centered on the health of the body, with a "joyful knowledge" that "we require for a new goal also a new means, namely, a new healthiness, stronger, sharper, tougher, bolder and merrier than any healthiness hitherto . . . "[5] This healthiness was not a state to be possessed complacently but rather one to be acquired again and again through an ongoing effort of will.

Seeing himself as a diagnostician of the spiritual sicknesses of his day, Nietzsche sought to uncover not only the ways in which the body and spirit had been split asunder, but also possibilities for becoming different, for transformation and creativity.[6]

This diagnostic approach is phenomenological[7] in that it advocates a direct experience of this split as a prelude to analyzing one's potential for change. No longer satisfied with a distanced, objective stance toward philosophical and scientific inquiry, the phenomenological perspective, beginning with Nietzsche and culminating in the movement in Europe known as phenomenological psychology, which we shall explore in Chapter 4, focuses on the subjective experience of the phenomena of one's own life.

Applying the phenomenological vision to human nature, Jung stressed the need to rediscover the body, too long a prisoner of the spirit, and to "reconcile ourselves to the mysterious truth that the spirit is the life of the body seen from within, and the body, the outward manifestation of the life of the spirit—the two being really one."[8]

Any therapeutic approach that seeks to integrate the psyche and body processes must help people gain a greater awareness and deeper physical experience of their ways of being in and reacting to the world.

Such awareness takes the form of a *bodily felt sense*[9] in which we feel ourselves to be inside ourselves, confronted with our deepest desires, wants, needs, dissatisfactions. Having achieved this awareness, we find it possible to "retrieve, from the very depth of our pain, our affliction, our . . . dissatisfaction, an experience of Being in its more hospitable, more wholesome dimensionality."[10] David Levin, a modern phenomenologist, terms this therapeutic process a *recollection*. It enables one not only to gain contact with and retrieve a sense of body-mind integrity and unity, but also to develop and cultivate the possibilities that stem from this bodily awareness. Once one has achieved a bodily felt sense of being in the moment, in the world—has achieved acute physical awareness of being *stuck* in a rigid frame of mind and of the rigidities of the body as they parallel and coexist with this mental rigidity—a variety of possibilities for change open up. In this sense, healing the body/mind split consists of recalling "what we were *given* to understand all along."[11]

The recollections of being of which Levin speaks are exemplified by the openness of vision experienced by the infant, who sees, feels, hears, and experiences the world, and his relationship to it, immediately and without preconceptions, without mediation by the ego and the critical functions. Experiencing, even for a moment, the infant's feeling of power enables us to realize that "what is today called 'healthy' represents a lower level than that which under favorable circumstances *would be healthy*—that we are relatively sick."[12]

From a somewhat different perspective, J. R. Worsley, founder of an English school of Five Element acupuncture[13] echoes Nietzsche's and Levin's purpose here, stressing that the goal of his form of acupuncture therapy is to help the client move beyond the relativity of the sickness or complaint by sensing *what he or she would be like when healthy*, when more completely whole, in body, mind, and spirit.

In working to heal the body/mind split by focusing on a state of being that *would be healthy*, we must learn to decipher the source of the psychological and physical blocks by reading the effects they have had on the body. This is like becoming aware of the effects of rain on soil erosion, or the effects of wind on the growth pattern of trees. Upon observing tight, hunched-up shoulders, for example, one might wonder to what extent this reflects the means, learned early in life, of coping with pressures and responsibilities. What is the connection between low backache and the feeling of carrying the weight of the world on one's back? Removing a wayward vertebra surgically may resolve a local problem, but it bypasses a bodily felt sense of the pressures of life. Only a *recollection* as described above can lead a person to straighten up and face life more healthfully. From a therapeutic perspective, recalling the effects of life's cares is equivalent to looking, historically, at the effects of the past on the present state of the body-mind, perceiving the *lived life*[14] of the bodymind.

If we were to stop at this first step in the therapeutic process, recognizing and treating the effects of life on the bodymind, we would already have accomplished a great deal. For as soon as one realizes how specific events, pressures, stresses, and emotional states have led to bodily changes, the reality of the total interconnectedness between mind and body becomes apparent, and the body/mind split has been mended. Simultaneously, however, the therapeutic approach alluded to above would take another step, utilizing the occasion of this bodily felt sense to grasp what could have been and what still can be. For example, after realizing that by adopting a "grin and bear it" attitude toward life's pressures one has developed chronic tension in the muscles of the shoulder and neck, it becomes possible to begin changing one's attitudes, ultimately freeing up a vast amount of energy hitherto deployed in the creation of a blockade against life in these muscles.

Levin stresses that a bodymind recollection is not only a *discovery* of what has been but also an *invention* or *creation* of what can be. But such therapeutic creativity will never occur if the therapist or doctor is also caught in the body/mind split.

Nowhere is this split more evident than in the education of doctors, psychologists, and other health and mental health care professionals.

From the very beginning it is implied in medical students' training that they should deal only with the physical body and its discrete parts. The initial trauma felt in dissecting a human cadaver rapidly gives way to a cold, detached, defensive posture that leaves little room for the cultivation of more human emotions. "The reality of dissection could not be endured," David Hilfiker tells us of his own medical training, "so we protected ourselves from it, built barriers between ourselves and the existence of our cadavers."[15]

Medical students have little time to ponder the meaning of life and death, so it is no surprise that they quickly learn professional mannerisms and sterile jargon which help them avoid such reflections. Little attention is paid in the student's curriculum to the teaching of interpersonal skills, which are so essential to those working with the ill, the troubled, and the bereaved. As a result, the patient often gets clinical detachment instead of human sensitivity.

On the other hand, the psychology intern is immersed from the outset in the realm of the imaginary. One course in neurophysiology is all this student is likely to get. Little wonder, then, that any physical complaint expressed by the client, once determined by a medical doctor to have no organic basis, will be perceived by the intern as imaginary, as only psychological. Ill-equipped by their education to understand the physical component of most complaints, psychologists learn to look through the body, into the mind of the client, thereby ignoring the physical aspect of the disorder.

Recently an airline stewardess came to see me with stomach complaints. If this woman had entered a physician's office, complaining of loss of energy and appetite, bloating beneath the waist, and general malaise following a recent flight, she would have undergone various physical and laboratory examinations aimed at detecting any pathologic condition in the gastrointestinal tract. If nothing abnormal had been discovered, she would have been so informed and dismissed. She might have left the office feeling relieved that the physician found nothing organically wrong, or she might have felt helpless and annoyed that while her complaint remained, she had been told that it had no objective basis. If she had returned a few days later, or after subsequent flights and told the physician that she felt unwell—adding that she, like many stewardesses she knew, suffered from "sagging internal organs," the physician might have referred her to a psychiatrist or psychologist who, having verified the physician's diagnosis of an absence of organic disorder, would have assumed the problem to be merely "in her head." He would have worked to help the patient express her feelings about flying, about her career, about her relations, and so on. In neither case would the woman's bodymind complaint have been seen as a living event, in its phenomenological entirety. She would thus have been forced to split her psychological and emotional experiences from experiences actually felt in the body.

An acupuncture therapist, on the other hand, would listen to, look at, and feel this woman's complaints in an entirely different fashion, concentrating on perceiving patterns that make sense of these various complaints and tie them together. From an acupuncture standpoint, a weakness would be seen in the spleen-organ energetic functioning, which is said, in ancient Chinese medical texts, to "hold up the internal organs and prevent prolapses." Some practitioners may also wish to explore the relationship between these complaints and the Earth element in traditional acupuncture theory. By constantly leaving the Earth (the Earth being associated with Spleen energetics) to go to foreign lands, stewardesses do weaken their internal organ functions. The sensation expressed by many stewardesses of a sagging in their internal environment would be taken quite seriously by an acupuncture therapist, or any body worker or psychotherapist attuned to the bodymind as an integrated unit.

One of the immediate benefits of acupuncture therapy is that it lends credence to the patient's *bodily felt awareness* and helps foster a *recollection of being* that is always a recollection experienced in the body and via the psyche.

Experienced medical doctors, despite knowing better, are obliged in most cases to act as if only a body and its parts were there in the office, because they possess few if any therapeutic techniques for intervening at the level of the psyche.

Likewise, most psychiatrists, clinical psychologists, and psychotherapists act as if only the psyche were in need of attention, and therefore view physical complaints as either a concern for the general practitioner or as data that must be interpreted for their psychological significance only.

While there is currently a movement in medicine toward understanding bodymind interaction, it has thus far remained in the realm of scientific research[16] and has not yet had any significant impact on the practice in our culture of molding either body doctors or mind doctors.

It is not a surprise, then, that patients routinely participate in this body/mind split and take only one part of their being to any particular practitioner.

The bodymind energetic approach, which will be developed in the following chapters, can be seen as a phenomenological approach aimed at helping people regain contact with their inner bodily awarenesses and potentials for change, by helping them become aware of their own body/mind splits and working with them on reintegration of the psyche and the body process.

BODY CURRENTS

Just as there is no adequate concept in modern medicine and psychology for an integration of mind and body, there is no place for a concept of human energetics and the forces that constitute human life.

While some physicists have been critical of modern medicine both for this omission and for remaining bound to the body/mind dualism despite the advances of modern physics, the orthodox medical view has demonstrated a striking resistance to, or inability to incorporate into its science, the knowledge of energy at the core of modern quantum physics.[17]

Modern medicine is not merely devoid of a philosophy of energy; it is, as Andrew Weil states, "glaringly deficient in theory and philosophy of any sort."[18] Seeing themselves as scientists, modern physicians need not be concerned with a philosophy of life or spiritual issues. Though they are sometimes discussed casually, feeling, thought, belief, and emotion are not given scientific credence. This is a serious omission, for a physician who does not take account of the psychological and spiritual lives of patients is never going to be able to practice, let alone teach, preventive medicine.

However, the picture may not be as desolate as it appears, for we are at a critical point where a new paradigm of health and healing aimed at preventive medicine and health maintenance is being established by a dedicated group of physicians, scientists, and therapists of body and mind.

This new breed of therapist and physician is interested in the possibility of a field theory in healing, informed by an appropriate concept of bodymind energetics that serves to connect physiology with spirituality. These practitioners share a vision of reality with modern physics, biology, and psychology, that, as Fritjof Capra, himself a physicist, informs us, "comes very close to the view of mystics and of many traditional cultures, in which knowledge of the human mind and body and the practice of healing are integral parts of natural philosophy and of spiritual discipline."[19]

Dr. Julian Kenyon, a British physician and researcher on electrical energy, holds that the most important phenomena for medical research and inquiry are energetic in nature. Starting from the premise that all biological events consist of electrical changes that can be detected by a variety of electricity-sensitive devices, much before any structural abnormalities have occurred, Kenyon underscores the importance of this understanding for preventive medicine. "If pathological changes can be detected at the energetic stage, then diagnosis can be much earlier, and also pathology at this stage is more easily reversible than when a lump has already appeared."[20] Unfortunately, the medical profession, with its emphasis on biology and biochemistry, views this idea with great skepticism. If doctors were trained more like physicists, Kenyon suggests, this energetic view would clearly appear to be the more scientific.

Dr. Robert O. Becker, an orthopedic surgeon who has devoted more than twenty years to research on limb regeneration and electrical forces in human beings, echoes Kenyon's remarks.

Returning to the vitalist concepts of the eighteenth century, most notably in the work of Galvani, Becker rediscovered the importance of electricity as the vital element in the life process. Beginning with the investigation of why and how salamanders are able to regenerate severed limbs, Becker and his colleagues have raised hard questions about the inability of humans to regenerate in the same fashion.

Against formidable obstacles presented by the scientific establishment, Becker continued his research; his discoveries led to a concept of electromagnetics in all living beings. In human beings, this constitutes a veritable *bio-electric self*, with great capacities for self-healing.

His work has contributed to the technique, now widely utilized, of bone-fracture healing by means of electrical stimulation, and continues to raise questions about the body electric—the body as a force field traversed by the same dynamic forces animating all of life.

With the advent of penicillin in the late 1920s, the transformation of medicine into a modern technology was complete. Whereas previously medicine had been an art combining the intuition and skills of the physician in making use of natural remedies proven effective over hundreds of years of experimentation, technological medicine adopted the position of a science—specifically, biochemistry—rather than an art.[21] The result of this technological shift, Becker maintains, is that medicine has lost its humanity.

Armed with the belief that medical practice is scientific, and that the effect of the therapies resides in the scientifically effective nature of the medications and procedures, the modern physician neglects the role played by personality in the treatment process and makes no use of the patient's innate healing capacity. "There's no need for the patient's own self-healing force nor any strategy for enhancing it. Treating life as a chemical automaton means that it makes no difference whether the doctor cares about—or even knows—the patient, or whether the patient likes or trusts the doctor."[22]

The result of the technological treatment of parts rather than patients, or symptoms rather than the person in all his or her complexity, is that many, including even those who can bear the incredible costs of these technological advances, feel estranged from modern medicine, leading to a paradoxical situation in which people avoid establishment medicine in favor of seemingly holistic (albeit often prescientific) modes of therapy that fail to appreciate the major advances of technological medicine. Disaffected patients are attracted to these alternative therapies, despite little scientific evidence of their efficacy, because there is a place in them for the *"doctor-patient relationship, preventive care,* and *nature's innate recuperative powers."*[23]

By placing all its eggs in the biochemistry basket, medical science has sacrificed the possibility of viewing medical phenomena from alternative perspectives. It has ignored the advances of a vitally alive physics with its promise of a field theory. While modern medicine appears to ignore these issues, the general public is beginning to become aware, explaining the popularity a decade ago of Capra's bestseller, *The Tao of Physics,*[24] which explores the relationship between Eastern mysticism and the new physics. Several new titles appear each year on this topic, and many speak about the human side of physics, about physics as a science as well as a way of viewing life.[25]

More people are turning toward Eastern philosophies and practices in which the concepts of life force and energy are present in ways that complement notions that appear in modern physics.[26]

These alternative views allow for a new paradigm in medicine that *problematizes* disease in a totally different way. Rather than concerning itself exclusively with the detection and treatment of organic disorders, the new paradigm, slowly expanding beyond the confines of the alternative medical world to the fringes of orthodox medicine, will direct itself toward the client's energy. Such a position leads to a collaboration among therapists of the body and the psyche, and raises questions about the possibility of early detection of energetic imbalances before any organic changes have occurred.

It could be said that the medical doctor never really diagnoses the *living event* of the patient's actual state of being and usually can arrive at a diagnosis for a condition only after it has taken months, years, or even decades to develop.

For example, a man in his forties diagnosed as having prostatitis may have spent years complaining to his doctor of low backache and dribbling urination. These complaints may well have been dismissed for years as insignificant when tests resulted in negative findings. Had this man's situation been assessed energetically or measured electrically at the outset, preventive treatment could have been initiated and prostatitis avoided.

Such vague complaints as these constitute from fifty to eighty percent of a general physician's practice. A premise of the new paradigm will be that if a patient feels something is wrong, then something really is out of balance and requires some sort of bodymind reintegration. Therapies will be judged no longer on the basis of their scientific validity alone, but rather in terms of how effective they are in understanding and treating the problem, as the patient experiences it.

This book will examine the energetic view of the body from two angles: first, from the ancient acupuncture-energetic perspective, which goes far toward explaining and treating many precise patterns of imbalance; and second, from the viewpoint of classic and modern psychosomatics, based on a conception of psychic energies. The result will be termed the "bodymind energetic" approach, which views the bodymind as an energetic phenomenon.

PSYCHOSOMATICS RETRIEVED

In a seminar I presented at an acupuncture conference three years ago, on the relationship between acupuncture and psychosomatics, those present showed little interest in acupuncture as a psychosomatic therapy. At a similar conference two years later, five of the lecturers emphasized the psychosomatic perspective. It therefore appears that the issue of psychosomatics has gained a certain urgency, and a purpose of this book is to provide the philosophical underpinnings for an approach that will combine psychosomatics and acupuncture energetics.

For the newly emerging bodymind paradigm to which this book

hopes to contribute, the focus will be less on diagnosis and treatment of disease, which will always be the province of medicine, and more on detection of energetic imbalances and on therapies of psyche and soma capable of intervening at the energetic level. A pragmatic series of interlocking psychological and somatic therapeutic models, and collaboration among therapists and physicians, will be advocated.

From such a perspective scientific precision in labeling disease will lose its position of importance and be replaced by a philosophical approach that places human beings within the context of their position in society and the universe. The new therapists and physicians agree with Georg Groddeck, the father of psychosomatics and the inspiration for the bodymind energetic approach, that "errors are not infrequently due to the striving after exactness in naming diseases, and that a different type of diagnosis will be developed which will not be satisfied with names, nor even with the findings made by examining the patient, but which will attempt to understand his situation in regard to his environment."[27]

ACUPUNCTURE, THE MISSING LINK

In contributing to a new perspective on psychosomatics, acupuncture energetics will be viewed as a missing link in the Western understanding of body and mind interactions. For more than two thousand years, Oriental physicians observed and recorded the ways in which symptoms of an imbalance occur along related energetic pathways known as meridians. This knowledge serves to explain relationships between what, in medical and psychological understanding, appear to be separate phenomena. Commonly in acupuncture treatment a therapist explains to the client how all of the symptoms are part of a particular energetic pattern, and receives eager confirmation from the client of a persistent feeling that the disparate symptoms were in fact connected. Acupuncture energetic patterns have been proved clinically, and treated for thousands of years successfully.

The inclusion of acupuncture energetics in the study of bodymind interaction will help us achieve the following aims.

First, this book hopes to convince Western acupuncturists of the necessity of moving beyond the traditional Chinese medical model in their studies, teaching, and practice of acupuncture, in order to develop new forms of acupuncture therapy specific to the issues confronted by Western clients. Remaining confined by the limits inherent in ancient Chinese medicine will artificially restrict the use Westerners can make of acupuncture both as a therapy and as an aid in reconceptualizing the relationship between mind and body. Ted

Kaptchuk notes that the Chinese model of healing, like Western medicine, is indeed a medical model focusing on the diagnosis and treatment of diseases, and that it is important for us in the West to advance away from the Chinese model of treating diseases, focusing
instead on maintaining health and well-being. In this sense we hope
that this book will serve as an aid in framing "the declaration of independence of Western acupuncture."[28]

Second, this book aims to demonstrate to body workers who deal
in the realm of what I shall term *somatic energetics* the importance and
usefulness of psychosomatics and acupuncture energetics. This will
enable them to direct their body work at an energetic level that does
not ignore the role of the psyche.

Third, this book sets out to restore interest in the psychoanalytically inspired work in psychosomatics done in the 1920s to the 1950s,
in order to provide psychotherapists no longer familiar with this
groundbreaking work, as well as acupuncture therapists and bodyworkers, with a phenomenology of psychic energetics that, unlike ancient Oriental philosophy, resonates with our own culture. The major reason for the relative disappearance of this work is its inability
to treat effectively the psychosomatic disturbances it analyzed so brilliantly. It was the vain hope of these therapists that modern physiology, and specifically endocrinology, would explain the often puzzling
relationships between certain emotional states and specific organ functions such as grief and asthma with accompanying constipation, which
the analyst could explain symbolically but not physiologically.
Acupuncture energetics, with its complex system of energetic connections relating specific organ functions with precise affective states, goes
far toward providing explanations for many hitherto undefined somatic reaction patterns and bodymind interrelationships. But to render the acupuncture perspective more useful in the treatment of Western bodymind disorders, we must also look to insights in Western
psychosomatics. Many who have shown an interest in Oriental philosophy and practices in the West suffer from a romanticism that ac-
cepts Eastern concepts unquestioningly. The wholesale adoption of
an Eastern mode of thought will not aid the development of a new
Western paradigm of health; the Asian medical models, as we shall
see, do not possess sufficient psychological theory to take into account
the psychology of the Western individual.

In this context, the myths and metaphors discovered by psychoanalysis and psychology match more closely our actual lived experience
than do the observations of Oriental "psychology."[29]

It should be noted that in advocating a combined use of the psychosomatic and acupuncture energetic perspectives, I do not subscribe
to the whole of the psychoanalytic approach. This book will be con-

cerned solely with that portion of the psychoanalytic oeuvre, from Groddeck on, that deals with the genesis of psychosomatic disorders, and the intricate relationship between psyche and soma in many, if not most, complaints. One need not agree with the psychoanalytic concepts of psychosexuality, leading to rigid sexual interpretations that reduce all events to a reliving of early family dynamics, to admire the philosophical precision and meticulous observation with which body-mind phenomena were perceived by the pioneers of psychosomatic medicine.

Finally, this book hopes to provide an image of bodymind energetics that will help lay readers recognize their own experience of their body and psyche, in order to restore the primacy of the subjective aware-ness of the client as central to any new bodymind therapeutics. Where the dominant medical system requires people to separate their men-tal and physical complaints, the bodymind phenomenological perspec-tive will argue in favor of a unified view of the bodymind, and a ther-apeutic process in which clients learn anew how to recollect how the bodymind would be were it unblocked and free-flowing.

In brief, this book sets out to develop a phenomenological approach to bodymind energetics, where the bodymind is seen as a complex energy field. In this fashion it resurrects the will or soul of therapist and client alike, as the active agent in the struggle to maintain health and prevent disease.

The new therapists will view the bodymind as a living, open sys-tem connected at all levels of its functioning to the heavens (cosmic energies, weather, influences of the sun and moon) and the earth (eco-logical and societal energies and forces). Such therapists will move beyond the mechanistic philosophy of Descartes and look to other areas where the issue of a field theory is being elaborated.[30]

The relativity of living systems, as energetic force fields, has parallels with ancient Chinese philosophy. Traditional acupuncture energetics, based on these ancient concepts of energy flow and transformation, will prove especially valuable in moving energetic therapies into the arena of human field theory.

In addition to the relativity of forces in relation to each other, one must take account of the relativity of one's own position as an ob-server and actor.

THE BODYMIND CONTINUUM

While conceptualizing the bodymind as an integrated unit is not new, Western practitioners and clients alike must learn to recognize their own relative position, be it closer to the *side of the psyche* (mind) or closer to the *side of the soma* (body) — and at the same time learn to appreciate other positions along what might be termed the *bodymind continuum*.

One client seeking help for a stiff neck may, in the initial consultation, begin to discuss the pains in his life, the disappointments and frustrations, the burdens, the traumas. Clearly, such a client is closer to the side of the psyche in his own bodymind experience of the world than is a client who comes in with the same problem, and is able to pinpoint with accuracy the precise vertebra involved and the nature and duration of the pain. Likewise, one practitioner will focus more on the nature of the body in question, noting posture, muscular rigidity or weakness, cold and hot areas of the the body, moving closer to the side of the soma than a practitioner who notes instead the content of the client's story and the inner workings of the emotions and the drives.

A working hypothesis of the discussion to follow is that we are all situated somewhere on the bodymind continuum, but that we are often very unclear about our position and at times behave negatively or critically toward those who occupy other positions on the spectrum.

Just the other day, for example, my ten-year-old son asked whether, if one had the choice, one would rather be the best athlete or the smartest pupil in school. The question shows that, already feeling the burden of the relative importance young boys assign to being good at sports, he was becoming aware of his and his parents' own positions on the continuum, closer to the side of the psyche. Suspecting that, given the absolute choice, we would favor intelligence (mind) over athletic ability (body), my son was struggling with how and where to situate himself. I hope he will not be caught in an absolute position that denies sports in favor of intellectual development alone, but rather will decide on the basis of his own strengths and preferences where to situate himself, without developing biases against children who occupy other positions on the bodymind continuum.

The Western mind works to a great extent by binary oppositions:[31] light and dark, good and evil, subject and object, inner and outer. Mind and body is simply another set of oppositions useful in making sense of the world around us and in ascertaining our relationship to it. However, it is essential for those working in health and mental health care to learn, for our own development as well as that of our clients, to recognize our own *relative* position while valuing other positions. We must see, within those positions furthest from our own, a major challenge for further development, rather than positions to be denounced as invalid. For the forming of binary oppositions, without an underlying sentiment of relativity, ultimately leads to the adoption of the most archaic opposition, namely Good and Evil. We must learn to do away with these prejudicial oppositions by relativizing our approach to health, well-being and illness. The issues involved are too complex to allow for absolute positions.

Below is a schematic of the Bodymind Continuum with some logical consequences that follow from each absolute pole on the continuum. It must be recognized that few of us ever occupy one absolute pole, but rather are situated somewhere in between.

SIDE OF THE PSYCHE	SIDE OF THE SOMA
PSYCHOsomatic Pole	SOMATICpsychic Pole
mind	body
long-term therapy	short-term therapy
getting to the "core"	seeing any problem as a reflection of the core
less visible	more visible
unmanifest	manifest
never focusing on symptoms	beginning with symptoms
working in depth	beginning at the surface
dependency	superficiality

Pushed to extremes, working from the PSYCHOsomatic side will tend to lead to more dependence of the client on the therapy, while working absolutely from the SOMATICpsychic side will tend to be superficial or even solely symptomatic. One goal of this book is to encourage us to move out of such absolute positions and learn to respect the complexity of the bodymind continuum.

A psychotherapist trained in psychoanalysis, who occupies a position far to the left on the continuum, might well assume that the core of a client's problems can only be reached slowly, over a long period of time, and will work with the client "in depth" to get to the underlying causes rather than concentrate on symptoms. Such a therapist might be very critical of a psychotherapist occupying a position further to the right, who works short-term, focusing on the client's main complaint and viewing it as a microcosm of deeper conflicts and issues. The latter often utilizes massage and breathing techniques to help clients feel their psychic conflicts somatically. The goal would be for the first therapist to work toward appreciating positions further toward the SOMATICpsychic pole, while the second therapist would learn to value positions further toward the PSYCHOsomatic pole. Such an appreciation might lead to learning somatic techniques if one works mainly from the side of the psyche and, conversely, learning counseling techniques to supplement one's bodywork; or it might lead to a referral network of like-minded body workers and psychotherapists who would collaborate in treating all sides of the bodymind complex in their clients. We trust that the reader will persevere in the pages to follow, reading somatic discussions with special care if tending more toward the side of the psyche and psychological discussions with more attention if oriented closer to the side of the soma.

In Chapter 2 we shall present a summary of acupuncture energetics for the reader unfamiliar with these concepts. The relationship between personality and predisposition to disease within the context of Western acupuncture will be explored in Chapter 3; a summary of the core psychosomatic concepts and phenomenological psychology will be addressed in Chapter 4. In the second half of the book, we shall present a phenomenology of the various energetic systems of the bodymind.

This is a book of philosophy and a philosophy of therapeutics whose concepts derive from clinical practice, interactions with body workers and psychotherapists, and exchanges with teachers and students of acupuncture and other health professionals. The ideas presented here have not been proved through scientific experimentation. Rather, they have been experienced in the context of work with others, both colleagues and clients, who see the goal of bodymind therapy as an *affirmation* of the client's being, and the techniques of this therapy as *supports* for the client's will to change and grow.

NOTES

1. Andrew Weil, *Health and Healing*. Boston, Houghton Mifflin Co., 1983, pp. 67–68.
2. Cf. Max Scheler's argument in David Michael Levin, *The Body's Recollection of Being: Phenomenological Psychology and the Deconstruction of Nihilism*. London, Routledge & Kegan Paul, 1985, pp. 57–58.
3. For a more spiritual reading of Freud's concepts, see Bruno Bettelheim, *Freud and Man's Soul*.
4. *The Body's Recollection of Being*, p. 33.
5. Friedrich Nietzsche, *Joyful Wisdom* (translated by Thomas Common). New York, Frederick Ungar Press, 1960, p. 351.
6. *The Body's Recollection of Being*, pp. 17–19.
7. As quoted in Levin, ibid., p. 13.
8. Carl G. Jung, "The Spiritual Problems of Modern Man," in *Civilization in Transition* (translated by R. I. C. Hal). Princeton, Princeton University Press, 1964, p. 94.
9. A term coined by Eugene Gendlin in *Focusing*. New York, Bantam Books, 1981.
10. *The Body's Recollection of Being*, p. 53.
11. Ibid.
12. Friedrich Nietzsche, *The Will to Power* (translated by Walter Kaufmann and R. J. Hollingdale). New York, Random House, 1968, p. 430.
13. J. R. Worsley is founder and current president of the College of Traditional Chinese Acupuncture, Leamington Spa, England, and has been the teacher of an entire generation of American acupuncture therapists, most notably Robert Duggan and Dianne Connelly, who began a school in Columbia, Maryland five years ago according to Worsley's teachings.

14. Known as reconstructing the *life history* of the individual, in phenomenological and existential psychology, *from the individual's subjective point of view.*
15. David Hilfiker, M. D., *Healing the Wounds: A Physician Looks at His Work.* New York, Pantheon, 1985, p. 27.
16. Cf. the work of the Institute for the Advancement of Health, and its journal *Advances,* edited by Harris Dienstfrey, which focuses on bodymind interactions and the new field of psychoneuroimmunology.
17. Cf. Fritjof Capra, *The Turning Point,* Part I. New York, Bantam Books, 1983.
18. Andrew Weil, *Health and Healing.* Boston, Houghton Mifflin Co., 1983, p. 113.
19. Fritjof Capra, *The Turning Point,* p. 385.
20. Julian Kenyon, "The Segmental Electrogram: A Non-Invasive Early Diagnostic Scanning Technique." *British Journal of Holistic Medicine,* Vol. 1, No. 2, December, 1984.
21. Cf. Robert O. Becker and Gary Selden, *The Body Electric,* Introduction. New York, William Morrow and Co., 1985.
22. Ibid, p. 19.
23. Ibid, pp. 19-20, emphasis ours.
24. Fritjof Capra, *The Tao of Physics: An Exploration of the Parallels Between Modern Physics and Eastern Mysticism.* Boulder Colorado, Shambhala, 1975, revised edition, 1983.
25. Cf. especially, K. C. Cole's *Sympathetic Vibrations: Reflections on Physics as a Way of Life.* New York, Bantam Books, 1985.
26. Cf. especially, *Encounters with Qi: Exploring Chinese Medicine* by David Eisenberg, M.D., with Thomas Lee Wright, New York, W. W. Norton & Company, 1987.
27. Georg Groddeck, *The Meaning of Illness.* New York, International Universities Press, 1977, p. 137.
28. "Acupuncture in the West—A Discussion between Ted Kaptchuk, Giovanni Maciocia, Felicity Moir, and Peter Deadman." *The Journal of Chinese Medicine,* Number 17, Jan, 1985, Sussex, England, pp. 22-31.
29. This is not meant to disparage Chinese psychological and philosophical reflection on Man's relation to society and the Universe, as in ancient Confucian and Taoist texts or practices such as the *I Ching (Book of Changes).* We wish only to emphasize that such reflection, which coincides with the development of Oriental medicine, can never satisfy the need for constructing a modern psychological understanding of the Western "individual" and the split between psyche and soma inherent in the development of this individual. The Chinese view of unity points us on a different way, but the way we take must, necessarily, be a Western way.
30. For a fascinating discussion of this trend, and a critique of Cartesian body/mind dualism, see Capra, *The Turning Point,* Part I.
31. As compared with the Eastern mind, which focuses on nuances. Cf. *Culture and Self,* edited by Marsella, Devos and Hsu, Tavistock, New York, 1985, p. 13.

2

Acupuncture Energetics: A Living System's View

> Chinese medicine appears to us as total psychosomatic medicine grafted onto the cosmic and hereditary environment. This whole is seen entirely energetically.[1]
>
> Schatz, Larre, de la Vallée

PHILOSOPHICAL BASES

Acupuncture energetics is a term I use to designate the traditional Chinese view of functional systems of the bodymind. This view of functional, energetic systems and their interrelations portrays the body as a microcosm of the forces of the universe, with Man situated between Heaven (the sun and moon and the cosmos) and Earth. A dynamic series of energetic fluctuations, working on the human organism from above and below, constitutes the body as a living system. In the discussion that follows, we shall present basic acupuncture-energetic theory. This presentation will serve as an introduction for the uninitiated reader, as well as a summary, from a bodymind-energetic perspective, for the acupuncture therapist.

Acupuncture-energetic theory encompasses five areas:

1. YinYang and the Eight Guiding Criteria
2. The Five Phases
3. The Energetic Functional Units
4. The Manifestations of Energy
5. The Meridian Energetic Systems

Generally speaking, these five areas are like five different but overlapping files in a computer. Presented with a clinical case, the acupuncture therapist will pull up one of these files, for example the YinYang file, as an aid in ordering in a meaningful way the data presented by the client. The therapist will match the presenting signs and symptoms against information in this file, gaining a perspective on the possible pattern underlying the client's complaints. The therapist might have enough information at this point to proceed to a treatment plan, but more probably another file will be pulled up; ideally, all five will be used to sift through and make sense of the data presented by the client.

In looking at a case from the *YinYang perspective,* a practitioner categorizes a complaint according to its energetic qualities (weak or strong, acute or chronic, hot or cold, superficial or deep). The *Five Phase perspective,* on the other hand, enables the practitioner to determine the possible origin of a disturbance, in one of five energetic constellations (known, metaphorically, as Fire, Earth, Metal, Water, and Wood) as well as predict the possible effects of the current disturbance on other, related constellations. A comprehensive series of correspondences exists for each of these constellations, facilitating the acupuncturist's task in connecting apparently distinct symptoms and information to arrive at a comprehensive picture of the client's energetic imbalance. In sifting the client's data through the sieve of the *energetic functional units* (consisting of twelve organ-energetic functional systems and their interrelationships), the practitioner will look for abnormalities in these functional systems. Perceived from the vantage point of the *manifestations of energy,* the client's imbalance will be categorized as a relative disorder of energy, or of blood or fluid circulation, or as an emotional disturbance affecting the spirit. Finally, in measuring the client's situation against the *meridian energetic systems* (composed of twelve major and eight secondary channels for the circulation of energy, and their multiple branchings throughout the body) the acupuncture therapist will be able to determine which meridian system, and which acupuncture points, to treat first.

These five areas together constitute traditional Chinese energetic anatomy and physiology, which is entirely distinct from Western anatomy and physiology. Whereas the Western perspective is concerned with studying the precise structure and function of different physical and biochemical aspects of the organism, the Eastern energetic model focuses on the energetic effects of the various functions of the bodymind, viewed as a field of forces.

Western anatomy and physiology, deriving from the dissection of the dead body into ever smaller observable parts, understands the human organism as the sum of these different parts. Essentially mechanical and structural, the Western body is a complex machine whose separate parts must be made to function properly, or be replaced or removed.

Eastern energetic anatomy and physiology, on the other hand, portrays the body as a dynamic, functional, unified field driven by forces, identical to those at work in the universe. In this view, the body is different from the sum of its parts and consists of a relatively balanced set of forces.

While the Western view is scientific and physical, leaving no room for a philosophical discussion of the will or spirit or soul of the individual, the Eastern perspective is metaphysical, and delineates a different will or soul attached to each functional unit, the sum of which constitute the spirit of the bodymind.

The acupuncture-energetic descriptions of bodymind dynamics are strikingly similar to those that describe the psychosomatic syndromes. In speaking of "organ inferiority" and "target organ," the classic psychosomatic approach arrives at explanations, similar to those of acupuncture, for the selection of a person's specific organ-functional systems as the site for the later development of disorders and diseases. When the early psychosomaticians, whose work we will summarize in Chapter 4, speak of "organ neuroses," they are making observations very similar to those of Chinese physicians, who for centuries catalogued these "organ neuroses" as ways in which the bodymind reacts to internal and external stress. The benefit of the acupuncture-energetic model is that it defines links where the psychosomatic perspective (and Western physiology) see none, and goes on to delineate a comprehensive system of treatment for these organ-functional disturbances. Acupuncture-energetic connections will often make sense of hitherto undefined bodymind interactions, aiding the body worker and psychotherapist in their work.

While the following summary of acupuncture energetics may prove difficult at certain points for the non-acupuncturist, a genuine attempt should be made to grasp the basic concepts, as they will be referred to, in the discussion of specific disturbances, in Part Two of the book. This energetic perspective will also provide medical and mental health practitioners with a comprehensive network of bodymind correspondences that will prove invaluable as images for learning to view the bodymind energetically.

YINYANG AND THE EIGHT GUIDING CRITERIA

Chinese philosophy holds that all living things are composed of two complementary forces.

The *Yin* forces are those that sustain and conserve the organism, that are at rest and quiescent, that condense and concentrate. In short, they are forces that remain latent, waiting to be organized. They are the bodymind's potential.

The *Yang* forces, on the other hand, are forces that produce and set into motion; they are forces that cause transformation and change, that expand, break down, and disperse. That is to say, they are the organizing forces, the dynamic principle.[2]

Yin, then, corresponds to the female principle, to nourishment and generation, to introversion and centripetal movement, to responsiveness and a conservative stance, and also to the earth, the moon, the fall and winter, coldness, moisture and fluids, the interior, the lower and front regions of the body, and the right side. The tendencies of Yin movement are toward condensing, sinking, and submerging. The Yin functions store what Chinese medicine usually refers to as nourishing energy, which derives from food and air and supports the organism.

Yang corresponds to the male principle, which is active and defends

YIN AND YANG COMPARED

YIN FORCES	YANG FORCES
completing	producing
resting	acting
sustaining	changing
conserving	transforming
condensing	expanding
concentrating	dispersing
awaiting organization	producing organization
nourishing	protecting
responding	commanding
female	male
passive	active
centripetal	centrifugal
earth	heaven
moon	sun
fall	spring
winter	summer
cold	hot
moist	dry
fluid	fire
interior	exterior
lower	upper
front	back
right side	left side
stores nourishing energy	generates defensive energy
introverted	extroverted

the organism, to extroversion and centrifugal movement, to aggressivity and a demanding stance toward life, to heaven and the sun, spring and summer, heat and dryness, fire and brightness, the exterior and the upper, back, and left aspects of the body. Yang movement tends to rise and float to the surface. The Yang functions transmit, transform, and eliminate unessential substances, but store nothing. Nourished by Yin forces, the Yang forces flow to the surface to protect the bodymind against external invasions.

YinYang theory is a theory of relativity. In fact, Yin and Yang are not fixed types of force, but rather a framework for categorizing forces in which everything possesses both a Yin and a Yang aspect, in such a way that Yin may transform at its apogee into Yang and vice versa. Yin and Yang create, control, and transform each other. In the web of cosmic events there is a constant interplay of Yin and Yang forces and correspondences, with no apparent cause but rather continual movement and change.[3]

The Eight Guiding Criteria

Clinically, all phenomena experienced by the client may be categorized into Yin and Yang, and usually the YinYang framework is expanded for this purpose into the Eight Guiding Criteria or the Eight Principal Patterns, namely Yin and Yang, Interior and Exterior, Deficiency and Excess, Cold and Hot.

This expansion of YinYang into eight categories creates a "conceptual matrix that enables the physician to organize the relationship between particular clinical signs and Yin and Yang."[4] While *Yin and Yang* serve as the broad criteria for categorizing clinical data, they are further refined by the use of the additional guiding criteria.

Interior and Exterior, the first derivation of Yin and Yang, refers both to the location of a disorder (deep inside or on the surface of the body) and to the directions from and to which the disorder develops (coming from the outside or moving to the surface, coming from the inside or moving deeper). An interior condition is one that is chronic and insidious in its development, possibly including such internal gastrointestinal symptoms as nausea, vomiting, or changes in stools and urine. Interior conditions are generally endogenous and are brought about by unabated internal stress of an emotional and psychological nature, constituting true psychosomatic disorders. Exterior conditions, on the other hand, are acute and sudden; usually accompanied by aversion to cold, wind, or heat; and often associated with fever. These disorders are exogenous, and the atmospheric energies (wind, cold, heat, dryness, dampness) are thought to be major precipitating factors of exterior conditions.

Deficiency and Excess, yet another formulation of Yin (deficiency) and

Yang (excess), are categories for the relative quantity of force at work in a given individual at a specific point in time. Conditions of deficiency include such disorders as insufficient energy or blood or fluids, or hypoactivity of any body function, with weakness, pale complexion, shallow breathing, and pain that is relieved by pressure. In brief, "deficiency patterns are usually chronic in nature, and may be thought of as a clinical landscape that is sparsely composed, bleak and desolate."[5]

Excess conditions, on the other hand, include conditions of accumulation of energy, blood, fluids, or other substances (which are the basis for cysts and tumors), the penetration into the body of atmospheric forces (or, more precisely, the development of hyperactivity and stepped-up immune responses against foreign invasions) or general overactivity of any of the body's energetic functions. While a person suffering from a deficiency condition tends to be weak, tired, soft-spoken, and introverted, a person with an excess condition is loud, moves forcefully, breathes heavily and rapidly, and has pains made worse by the application of pressure. "In general, patterns of Excess tend to be acute, and may be seen in the mind's eye as a cluttered clinical landscape."[6]

The final YinYang formulation, *Cold and Hot,* is useful in describing the quality of an imbalance. Cold disorders show signs such as a slow pulse; fear of cold; lethargic, introverted movement; pain relieved by the application of heat; and a white tongue coating. The basic quality of a cold pattern "is 'cloudy,' like an overcast, frozen winter."[7] Heat patterns, on the other hand, are those with a rapid pulse, dislike of heat, agitated activity, extroversion, thirst, and a desire for cool climates. Heat patterns portray a quality that "is 'bright,' and its mood is 'jumpy'."[8]

Treatment Implications of the YinYang Approach

The treatment implications that follow from the YinYang approach lead to a more or less physical energetic therapy. The Eight Guiding Criteria help define the more manifest, more material nature of an energetic imbalance in physical terms (stuck blood, stagnant energy, accumulation of dampness). This way of viewing disorders, exemplified in the modern Chinese approach to acupuncture and herbology known as *Traditional Chinese Medicine,* is heavily influenced by a herbal perspective and bias that seeks to define precisely the material substances of the body as manifestations of energy. Such a perspective necessarily leads to treatment of physical symptoms with a selection of points that mirrors the disorder, and seeks resolution of these symptoms and complaints as one of the primary goals of therapy. This approach is

YINYANG AND THE EIGHT GUIDING CRITERIA

YIN	YANG
Interior	*Exterior*
Location of a disorder and direction from which it emanated or to which it is evolving	
Chronic, insidious in development, possible gastrointestinal symptoms, endogenous, prompted by internal stressors	Acute, aversion to cold, wind, heat, possible fever, exogenous, prompted by atmospheric conditions (wind, chill) and a lowered resistance
Deficiency	*Excess*
Quantity of force at a specific time and place	
Insufficiency of energy, blood or fluids, functional hypoactivity, pale complexion, weakness, shallow breathing, pain relieved by pressure	Accumulation of energy, blood, fluid (cysts, tumors), functional hyperactivity, loud, forceful behavior, heavy, rapid breathing, pain worsened by pressure
Cold	*Hot*
Quality of an imbalance	
Slow pulse, slow, lethargic activity, aversion to cold, pain eased by heat, white tongue coating, introverted	Rapid pulse, rapid, agitated activity, aversion to heat, thirst, desire for cool climate and drinks, red tongue, extroverted

best suited for *somatic energetic reaction patterns*, whereas the Five Phase approach, as we shall now see, may be more appropriate for treatment of what could be called psychoenergetic imbalances of body, mind, and spirit.

FIVE PHASES

While YinYang, and the Eight Guiding Criteria that derive from it, are extremely useful in categorizing the phenomenology of the body's dynamic interrelations, ancient Chinese philosophy provides yet another major organizing system, known as the theory of the Five Elements or Phases.

In this philosophical view, the Five Elements that constitute the material world are Fire, Earth, Metal, Water, and Wood. Together they constitute a framework for postulating a multiplicity of correspondences between the signs and symptoms manifested by a client. These correspondences, for example between the Fire phase and the summer, the heart function and emotional warmth, are part of a traditional belief system within Chinese philosophy that postulates a fundamental relatedness between Man and the cosmos. Critics of the Five Phase approach see it as a metaphysical, archaic set of beliefs but admit to its usefulness as a mnemonic device for learning how symptoms are connected in specific patterns in traditional Oriental medicine.

While many modern practitioners of acupuncture in the East have forsaken the Five Element perspective, it is impossible to speak of any energetic pattern of disharmony without utilizing correspondences and concepts that derive from the Five Phases and Elements.[9]

In the chart given here, we have summarized the principle correspondences between each Element, and the Yin and Yang organ-energetic functions that belong to it. The organ-energetic function of the Liver, for example, within the Wood Element, is related to the Gallbladder (its Yang-paired function), the sense of sight, the functioning of the muscles and tendons, the birth cycle in nature, the nails, tears, the rancid odor and sour taste, the sound of shouting, the color green, an angry or depressed disposition, wind, and the season of spring. To speak of a disturbance of the Liver organ-energetic function, then, might relate as readily to a problem with the muscles that tends to show up in the spring or after exposure to a draft (wind) as to a person who is alternately angry and depressed, with a greenish complexion and craving for sour foods.

We will look at the twelve major organ-energetic functional units in the next section, but it must be understood at this point that these functional units cannot be fully understood without knowing the Five Element correspondences that weave the fabric of any of the Five Phase constellations. Despite the antipathy of many modern practitioners to the metaphorical and metaphysical nature of the Five Element theory, the very nature of Chinese medicine, and especially acupuncture energetics, reveals the imprint of these Elements, whose material reality is readily grasped by a properly trained therapist.

While criticized heavily in modern China as a metaphysical system that has outworn its validity and usefulness in aiding clinicians in their daily work, the Five Elements and phase energetics have proven especially intriguing and clinically useful in the West. Perhaps this is because in the West, there is a loss of connection between Man and Nature, and the natural forces have come to be seen as mere tools in the service of humankind. Such a modern, technological view requires a contrasting, ancient view that respects Nature and its elemental forces.

Five Phase Correspondences

The Five Phases or Elements is a system that connects specific organ functions, as just stated, with a series of energetic correspondences, which we provide here in chart form. It must be borne in mind that these correspondences stem from thousands of years of clinical observation, and most are readily observable to the acupuncture therapist.

These series of correspondences, constituting the separate constellations of Fire, Earth, Metal, Water, and Wood Energetic Phases, are learned at the beginning of an acupuncture student's studies. Reference will be made to these correspondences in the rest of the book, so it is suggested that the reader become familiar with these correspondences or keep this chart marked for ready reference.

These correspondences are often seen in everyday life as well as in syndromes of traditional Oriental medicine. They are an invalu-

FIVE PHASES: SERIES OF CORRESPONDENCES

	Wood	*Fire*	*Earth*	*Metal*	*Water*
YIN organ fuction	Liver	Heart Pericardium	Spleen	Lungs	Kidneys
YANG organ function	Gallbladder	Small Intestine Triple Heater	Stomach	Large Intestine	Bladder
sense	sight	speech	taste	smell	hearing
tissue	muscles & tendons	blood vessels	flesh, body shape	skin	bones
cycle	birth	growth	transformation	harvest	storing
opens to	nails	complexion	lips	body hair	head hair
fluid	tears	sweat	saliva	mucus	urine
body odor	rancid	scorched	fragrant	fleshy	putrid
temperament	anger, depression	joy, volatile emotions	worry, sympathy	grief	fear
taste	sour	bitter	sweet	hot, spicy	salty
sound	shouting	laughing	singing	weeping	groaning
climate	wind	heat	dampness	dryness	cold
season	spring	summer	late summer	fall	winter
color	green	red	yellow	white	black

able aid in directing the attention of a practitioner toward salient features of a client's bodymind-energetic imbalances. For example, when interviewing a person who shows a tendency to shout out words, the practitioner would know this denotes an angry disposition and would be reminded to ascertain whether this person had disorders of vision, muscle spasms or twitches, deformed or cracked nails, an aversion to wind, and so forth, all of which point to the Wood phase. These Five Phase correlations are made automatically, even by the beginning student. While not always entirely accurate, they are usually very beneficial in drawing up a picture of the energetic disharmony. Therefore, the Five Phase correspondences teach a practitioner to widen the scope of observation, to include data not normally included in a medical or psychological evaluation, and thereby to learn to perceive the reality of energetics through the traces it leaves in the bodymind. These correspondences are a type of detection device for reading energetic movements and deciphering their phenomenological significance by fitting them into a pattern specific to the individual.

Energetic Cycles

The Five Phases are thought to constitute a system for understanding energetic physiology (the movement of energy through the various organ energetic functional units) and guide the practitioner in comprehending the energetic disturbances of the bodymind as well as explaining the etiology of these disturbances.

There are two normal cyclical energetic relationships, known as the generation and the control cycles.

1. *Generation cycle.* Starting with Fire, every phase is viewed as the "mother" of the following phase and the "child" of the preceding phase (e.g., Fire, as can be seen in the diagram, is the mother of Earth and the child of Wood).

In normal daily functioning, energy circulates along the generation cycle, from Fire to Wood and around again. There is thought to be a system of energetic physiological checks and balances, known as the control cycle, to control this daily circulation.

2. *Control cycle.* Every phase is thought to be controlled by one other phase and to control or check one phase in turn, in order to insure the normal energetic physiological circulation. The control cycle is illustrated in the diagram here where it can be seen, for example, that Fire controls Metal and is controlled in turn by Water, and Earth controls Water and is controlled by Wood, and so on.

The checking nature of the control cycle is such that an excess or hyperactivity of a phase will be kept in check by the normal physiological nature of the phase controlling it. For example, Wood is kept in check by Metal.

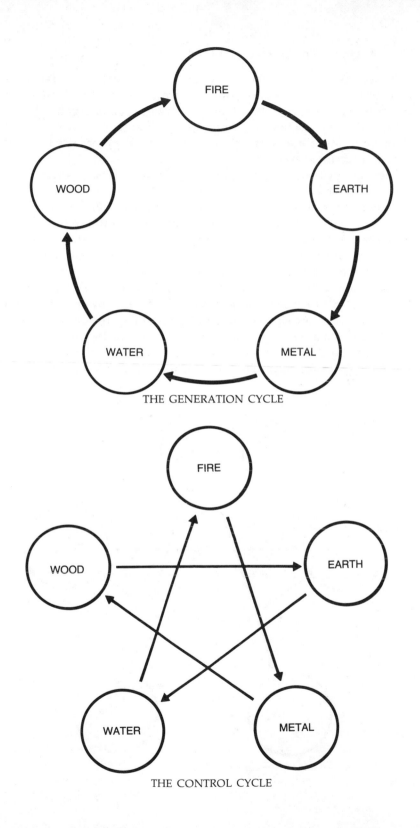

THE GENERATION CYCLE

THE CONTROL CYCLE

When a sufficient number of factors—such as external adverse climate or stress, or internal emotional turmoil, undernourishment, or inherited weaknesses—occur together, or when an energetic phase is disturbed in its functioning, these normal energetic controls may become injurious to the phases they keep in check, giving rise to pathological *reaction patterns.*

There are two such reaction patterns, known as the destruction cycle and the violation cycle.

1. *Destruction cycle.* This cycle follows the same order as the control cycle depicted. In a pathological situation, when a phase has become weakened or hypoactive, it is vulnerable to attack by the phase that normally controls it. For example, if the Earth phase becomes weakened or hampered in its functioning because of internal or external factors, then the Wood phase, whose normal energetic function is to keep the Earth phase in check, will instead begin to encroach upon and injure the Earth phase functions, providing the foundation on which illness may develop. In addition, if a phase becomes hyperactive, it may begin to harm the normal energetic functioning of the phase it is responsible for controlling. For example, if Earth is overly active,

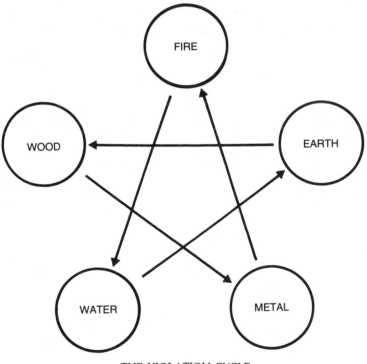

THE VIOLATION CYCLE

it may invade and harm the Water-energetic functions, the phase it normally controls. This might lead to disturbances in the salient organ-energetic functions, that of the Kidney and Bladder functions in this example.

2. *Violation cycle.* This cycle is a reverse of the destruction cycle. Here the function of a phase, if disturbed, may rise back up against its controller. For example, if the function of Fire is upset, it may do harm to its controller, Water. Thus a Water-energetic disturbance may result from this Fire imbalance. It is said that the disturbed function of Fire is violating or flowing back against the normal control of Water over Fire, as depicted here.

The normal and abnormal energetic physiological relationships of the Five Phases may be summed up using the Wood phase as an example, as follows:

1. Wood is the mother of Fire;
2. Wood is the child of Water;
3. Wood is controlled, under normal energetic conditions, by Metal, or injured, when Wood is imbalanced, by Metal;
4. Wood controls Earth, under normal conditions, and injures Earth under adverse conditions;
5. Wood, while normally controlled by Metal, may rise up against Metal under adverse conditions.

Treatment Implications of the Five Phase Approach

From the examples given here, it can be seen that action on any given phase has strong repercussions on the other phases with which it interacts. In treatment, therefore, the Five Phase approach is very powerful and far fewer needles are used—normally only a couple, as compared with the YinYang approach discussed earlier. This is because Five Phase treatment goes deeper than the energetic pattern of imbalance that the client may be suffering from at the moment, to effect a change at the root of this imbalance in whatever energetic phase is found to be disturbed. One needle placed in a point[10] on the Wood function of Liver, for example, might suffice to give more energy to the Fire function of the Heart and dispel the pathological effects of the Water function of the Kidneys on the Fire organ-energetic functions. Such treatment is very delicate and aims at harmony between body, mind, and spirit. It is more esoteric and spiritual, and less indicated in the resolution of specific somatic-energetic reaction patterns. The Five Phase approach, as we shall see in some detail in Chapter 3, is best suited for *psychoenergetic reaction patterns.*

Both the YinYang and the Five Phase approaches have their special

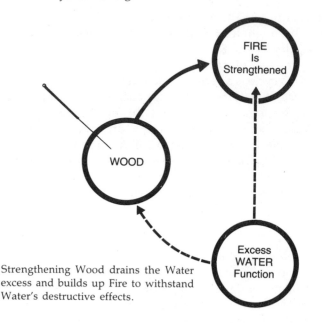

Strengthening Wood drains the Water excess and builds up Fire to withstand Water's destructive effects.

areas of application; it is a tribute to Western acupuncture that the integration of these two approaches is being accomplished, whereas the modern Chinese approach has all but forgotten or lost the older Five Phase modalities as well as the ability to intervene on a more psychological and spiritual level.[11]

THE ENERGETIC-FUNCTIONAL UNITS

A Western Liver Is Not a Chinese Liver

Chinese medical thought is primarily functional and dynamic, addressed at observing patterns of energetic relationships among physiological events. Thus, when the various organs are mentioned, they refer to energetic-functional units rather than, as is customary in Western medicine, to the somatic structures involved. For example, the organ called liver connotes something quite different in Chinese and Western medical terms, the former defining the liver by the energetic functions associated with it and the latter understanding it to mean a definite physical structure and its specific functions. "This divergence of conceptual approach makes it possible for Chinese medicine to identify Organs not recognized in the West—such as the Triple Burner—and not to recognize organs and glands clearly identified by Western medicine—such as the pancreas and the adrenal glands."[12]

While it is important to draw bridges between Western and Oriental concepts in order to facilitate communication between practitioners of both medicines, it must be borne in mind that any attempt to develop strict parallels between Oriental energetic and Western biochemical physiology and pathology will be inappropriate or misleading in many cases.[13]

Organ-Functional Units

In the Oriental medical model, there are twelve major organ-energetic functions or spheres of influence, six of them Yin and six Yang. The Yin organ-energetic functions are Heart, Pericardium, Spleen, Lungs, Kidneys and Liver. These Yin functions are related to the storing of vital essences and have to do with the generation, regulation, transformation, and storage of energy, blood, fluids, and spirit (*shen*). Yin functions are conceived of as deeper and more essential for vital functioning than the Yang functions.

The Yang organ-energetic functions are Small Intestine, Triple Heater, Stomach, Large Intestine, Bladder, and Gallbladder. These Yang functions are primarily active and relate to the breaking down of food and fluids and the absorption of nutrients from them, the circulation of the derived "nourishing energies" around the body, and the secretion of unused materials.

The organ-energetic functions are summarized here. The reader interested in more detail should consult the texts in the bibliography.[14]

YIN ORGAN-ENERGETIC FUNCTIONS AND DYSFUNCTIONS

	Energetic Functions	Energetic Dysfunctions
HEART	1) Rules over Blood and Vessels, promoting smooth blood flow and pulse and heartbeat.	1) Irregular blood flow, blood vessel disorders, irregular pulse and beats, all arrhythmias.
	2) Stores the Spirit (*Shen*), leading to regular behavior and adequate responses to the environment.	2) Irrational behavior, insomnia, excessive dreaming, hysteria, delirium.
	3) Opens to the tongue, governing tongue color and speech.	3) Pale or purple tongue, tongue ulcers, slurred speech, fast talking, speech defects.
	4) Shows in the complexion, rendering it normally ruddy.	4) Pale, lusterless complexion, purplish, congested complexion.
PERICARDIUM	1) Protector of the Heart, warding off external pathogenic influences to protect the heart energetic function.	1) Pericarditis; any disorder affecting the heart due to environmental or emotional stress.

YIN ORGAN-ENERGETIC FUNCTIONS AND DYSFUNCTIONS (continued)

	Energetic Functions	*Energetic Dysfunctions*
LUNGS	1) Directs descending (inhalation) and moistening movements.	1) Disorders of inhalation; dry skin, throat, nose.
	2) Directs circulating and disseminating (exhalation).	2) Disorders of exhalation, fluid accumulation, energy accumulations.
	3) Rules Qi (Energy); governs respiration.	3) Respiratory disorders and fatigue in general; low resistance.
	4) Moves the Waterways (liquids down to the Kidney function).	4) Edema, fluid retention, perspiratory disturbances, urinary disorders.
	5) Rules the Exterior (Skin, pores), leading to normal sweating and skin moisture.	5) Disorders of perspiration, dry skin, weak external defenses.
	6) Opens to the nose, throat, vocal cords.	6) Fluttering wings of the nose; dryness and scratching of the throat, voice disorders, weak voice projection.
	7) Manifests in the body hair.	7) Disorders affecting body hair.
SPLEEN	1) Rules over transportation and transformation (of food into blood and Qi.	1) Deficient Qi or Blood anywhere in the body, abdominal swelling, malabsorption, abdominal pain, loss of appetite, loose stools.
	2) Governs the Blood and maintains it in the channels.	2) Blood in vomit, stools, urine; all bleeding disorders.
	3) Governs muscle tone, flesh, and the extremities.	3) Poor muscle tone, fleshiness, weak or sluggish extremities.
	4) Opens to the mouth, manifests in the lips, leading to proper ability to taste and red moist lips.	4) Taste irregularities or insensitivity, pale or dry lips.
LIVER	1) Rules over smooth flow of Qi, leading to balanced body movement.	1) Stagnant blood or energy leading to pain and distention, swollen breasts, pelvic accumulations, cysts, lumps, erratic body movements.
	2) Controls bile secretion.	2) Digestive disturbances, bitter taste.
	3) Harmonizes the emotions leading to an even disposition.	3) Irritability, anger, frustration, angry depression, uneven disposition.
	4) Stores Blood.	4) Blood deficiencies, excess or deficient menstrual flow.

YIN ORGAN-ENERGETIC FUNCTIONS AND DYSFUNCTIONS (continued)

	Energetic Functions	*Energetic Dysfunctions*
	5) Governs tendons and muscles, leading to proper muscle movement; and manifests in the nails.	5) Disorders of the tendons, muscle spasms, thin brittle nails.
	6) Opens to the eyes.	6) Many eye and visual disorders, including spots in visual field, night blindness, visual disturbances of migraines, and so on.
KIDNEYS	1) Stores Ancestral Energy (*Jing*), the source of reproduction and growth and maturation.	1) Congenital disorders; reproductive, maturational, and developmental disturbances.
	2) Rules Water metabolism (with Lungs and Spleen).	2) Edema, water metabolism disorders, urinary disorders.
	3) Rules over bones and produces marrow.	3) Disorders of bones (stiff spine, weak legs and knees, brittle bones, low back disorders), poor teeth.
	4) Opens to the ears and manifests in head hair.	4) Hearing disorders, devitalized head hair, hair loss on head.
	5) Grasps Qi from the lungs, to promote moistening.	5) Respiratory disorders, coughing, asthma due to weakness.

YANG ORGAN-ENERGETIC FUNCTIONS AND DYSFUNCTIONS

	Energetic Functions	*Energetic Dysfunctions*
SMALL INTESTINE	1) Rules separation of pure from impure, hence food absorption with Yang function of the Spleen.	1) Abdominal pain and rumblings, diarrhea, constipation, malabsorption.
TRIPLE WARMER	1) Rules the three regions of the body (Head and Chest; Digestive Organs, Kidney & Reproductive Functions).	1) Disharmonies between the three regions or in one specific region.
	2) Controls the waterways (coordinates functions of Lungs, Kidneys, and Spleen).	2) Fluid metabolism and temperature disorders, edema.
LARGE INTESTINE	1) Moves impure food and fluids downward.	1) Abdominal pain, rumblings, intestinal disorders.
	2) Absorbs water from wastes.	2) Water and fluid deficiency, diarrhea, constipation.
STOMACH	1) Receives, rots, and ripens food.	1) Stomach pain, poor digestion, nausea, abdominal distention, belching, vomiting.

YANG ORGAN-ENERGETIC FUNCTIONS AND DYSFUNCTIONS (continued)

	Energetic Functions	*Energetic Dysfunctions*
	2) Intimately connected to Spleen, digestive functions.	2) All digestive disturbances.
GALLBLADDER	1) Stores and secretes bile.	1) Bile disorders, bitter taste, digestive disturbances.
	2) Works closely with Liver.	2) Liver organ functional disturbances.
BLADDER	1) Receives and excretes urine.	1) Urinary retention, incontinence, dribbling.
	2) Controls urination.	2) Urinary retention, incontinence, dribbling.

Organ-Energetic Pathophysiology

The Yin and Yang organ functions work in pairs, with one Yin and one Yang function interconnected. These six pairs fit within the Five-Phase Energetic model as follows:

YINYANG FUNCTIONAL PAIRS

Yin		*Yang*	*Phase*
Lung	paired with	Large Intestine	METAL
Spleen	paired with	Stomach	EARTH
Heart	paired with	Small Intestine	FIRE
Kidney	paired with	Bladder	WATER
Pericardium	paired with	Triple Warmer	FIRE
Liver	paired with	Gallbladder	WOOD

These six pairs of Yin and Yang organ-energetic functions can be depicted in the Five-Element circle, with the Yin organ energetic functions on the interior of the circle and the Yang functions on the exterior.

Energetically, each organ function has a *Yin* (storing, nourishing, cooling) component and a *Yang* (activating, protective, warming) component, stemming from the Yin and the Yang Roots of the Kidneys respectively. The Yin and Yang Roots represent the genetic inheritance from the parents—the energetic, organizing principle, the genetic code. According to acupuncture-energetic embryological theory, within the Yin (viscous, pure) potential of the egg, the first Yang (active) movement to take place is the appearance of that point (in what will be the lumbo-sacral region of the lower spine) known as *ming-men* or "gate of life." While the Yin of the Kidneys refers to the potential stored

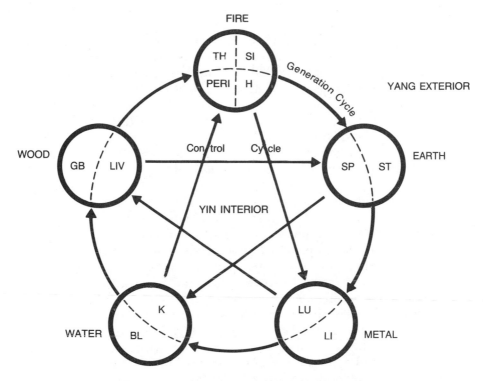

YINYANG FUNCTIONS AND THE FIVE PHASES

within the fetus, the Yang of the Kidneys refers to the spine and the active organization of the different parts and functions of the body as they emerge in the fetus. The Yin of the Kidneys is a term used to designate those energetic functions associated with reproduction, essence, the genetic code in general (i.e., pure potential), body fluids and their metabolism, and the cooling of the body. The Yang of the Kidneys, in turn, refers to those functions associated with body heat, sexual energy, the active functioning of the organism, the warming of the body. A tendency toward a relative deficiency of either the Yin or the Yang Root of the Kidneys may often be detected. This will affect the relative deficiency or excess, hypoactivity or hyperactivity of the associated Yin- or Yang-energetic functions. In a situation where the Yin Root is weak there will be a deficiency of Yin (body fluids and cooling action) with resultant dry skin and scalp; dry, red eyes; and disorders of rising heat (tinnitus, high blood pressure, conjunctivitus, hyperthyroidism, irritability, insomnia, and so forth). This is because with a deficiency of Yin, Yang functions and movement will be uncontrolled. Phenomenologically, one might term this phase the

Becoming Yang or *Becoming Hot* phase, to denote this unchecked rise in activity and heat.

The converse of this condition is a deficiency of the Yang Root of the Kidneys, resulting in an inability of the body to maintain proper body heat or burn up excess fluids, with an aversion to cold, cold regions in the body, slow metabolism, low blood pressure, mucus build-up, hypothyroidism, fatigue, and an accumulation of fluids (edema, water retention). This phase may be termed the tendency to a *Becoming Yin* or *Becoming Cold* state of functioning.

This simple schematization of the basic tendencies toward Yin or Yang functioning is very useful in understanding the possible disturbances a person may develop. If we situate the Yin of the Kidneys on the left side of the Five Phase diagram and the Yang of the Kidneys on the right side, we see that when the Yin of the Kidneys is deficient, "becoming hot" tendencies will develop in those organ-energetic functions on the left side of the diagram, namely within Wood and Fire, with rising heat disorders in the Liver, Gallbladder, and Heart, specifically. However, when the Yang of the Kidneys is deficient, "becoming cold" tendencies will take over, with cold disorders and a build-up of fluid and mucus occurring in those energetic functions on the right side of the chart, in Earth and Metal primarily, with cold in the Stomach, a decrease in the Yang aspects of the Spleen functions, and a build-up of mucus in the Lungs. This may be portrayed in chart form as shown at right:[15]

These two major dysfunctional tendencies will be referred to in Part II of this book, so the reader may wish to become familiar with this diagram, or keep it marked for ready reference later on.

MANIFESTATIONS OF ENERGY AND BODY SUBSTANCE

In acupuncture-energetic theory, the fundamental substances of the bodymind are divided into manifestations of *Qi* (Energy), *Blood, Fluids, Ancestral Energy,* and *Spirit.*

Qi is "matter on the verge of becoming energy, or energy at the point of materializing"[16] and is defined functionally as that which promotes movement in the bodymind, protects the organism (the function of protective or defensive energy), provides for various transformations (of food and fluids and Air into Qi, Blood, Fluids, tears, urine), retains Organ functions in their proper place (holding up Organs, especially in the abdominal area and below, and keeping Blood in its pathways) and warms the body.

Qi may also be defined by the area or zone it energizes, as Organ Qi, Meridian Qi, Nourishing Qi, Defensive or Protective Qi, and the Qi of the Chest.

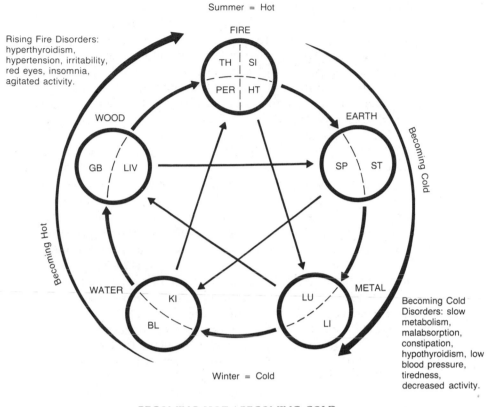

Summer = Hot

Rising Fire Disorders: hyperthyroidism, hypertension, irritability, red eyes, insomnia, agitated activity.

Becoming Cold Disorders: slow metabolism, malabsorption, constipation, hypothyroidism, low blood pressure, tiredness, decreased activity.

Winter = Cold

BECOMING HOT / BECOMING COLD

Qi may be deficient, leading to lethargy, pale face, weak voice, lack of desire to move, and a weak pulse. It may also be excessive because of stagnant energy in a specific Organ-energetic zone or area of the body, with resultant distention and pain, a purplish tongue, soft changeable lumps, and a wiry pulse.

Blood is a nourishing, liquid, Yin substance, similar to but not identical with the Western concept of Blood. It is essentially thought to be not only the red fluid that travels in the blood vessels, but also the nourishing (as opposed to protective) aspect of the energy that flows through the vessels.

Blood can be deficient and is associated with a thin, weak, emaciated constitution; dizziness; visual disturbances such as seeing spots or weakened vision; numbness of the extremities; general dryness; scanty menstruation; a pale face that is lusterless, and a thin pulse denoting an insufficiency of blood to fill the vessels and arteries. Blood may also be congealed in a specific organ function or zone of the body.

This condition is accompanied by stabbing pain; relatively hard, stationary lumps or tumors; a darkened complexion; a dark purple tongue, at times exhibiting red spots; and a rough "choppy" pulse.[17]

Ancestral Energy (Jing) is the congenital, constitutional potential inherited from one's parents and includes the genetic code determining all growth processes throughout life. It is the basis of reproduction and development, and is replenished during life by the pure aspects derived from air, food, and water. Disorders due to a deficiency of Ancestral Energy include any congenital defects or inherited predispositions to disease ("organ inferiorities") as well as disorders of maturation and growth.

Spirit (Shen) is the vitality of the individual, that which constitutes him or her as this person and no other, the very force that infuses the personality. A person with spirit is one whose force is clearly deployed and keenly felt by others. Oriental energetic physiology postulates that each Organ function has a particular character or spirit all its own, constituting the "twelve officials."[18] It is here, in the concept of spirit as a particular force taking shape in each zone and function of the bodymind, that acupuncture energetics demonstrates a fundamental psychosomatic perspective. For example, the spirit of the Liver-energetic function has to do with vision and foresight (the Liver meridian travels to the eyes), the ability to plan, to keep calm and display a smoothness of emotions, and to act in the external world with creativity and an openness to change. While this anthropomorphization or personification of organ function may strike the reader as peculiar, we in the West have always thought this way too, as can be seen in such expressions as a "bilious temper" or a "disorder of Spleen" or a "heartbreaking" event or a "liverish disposition." In the movement of Western medicine from metaphysics to science, the notion of a spiritual aspect of the body and its functions fell into disfavor, as did the notion of a vital force driving the organism. All discussion of such matters was left to the emerging sub-field of psychiatry, where, unfortunately, the issue of the actual physicality and real functional nature of the spirit or psyche and its activity was sidestepped by talk of psychological and spiritual life as an unreal, imaginary realm. While Western medicine reserved a place within itself—in this sub-field that has never been totally adopted as a full-fledged field of medicine—for study of the spiritual nature of psychic life, it did so in a radically disembodied way. Henceforth, physical complaints were seen as "real" and psychical complaints as "imaginary." This body/mind split is still at work in most areas of medicine, despite the spread of psychotherapy.

One trend—classic psychosomatics, which we shall study in some detail in Chapter 4—developed a way of talking about the material reality of the psychic nature of the organ functions by talking of "organ" or "vegetative" neuroses. These psychic organ-functional disturbances bear a surprising similarity to the organ-energetic dysfunctions of acupuncture energetics, and the combination of these two perspectives, in the bodymind-energetic approach proposed here, will infuse both perspectives with more force for bringing the reality of the unity of bodymind functioning into the center of the new paradigm of health that is emerging in this country. It is impossible to adopt a sterile, detached attitude toward body dysfunctions once one attributes a spiritual or psychic dimension to them. Disturbances of Spirit or *shen*, in the acupuncture framework, will denote what we in the West would term behavioral, emotional, and psychological disorders.

Fluids in the acupuncture-energetic system are the same as in Western physiology: sweat, saliva, gastric juices, urine, blood, serous fluid—all the fluids of the body that moisten it and keep it from overheating. A deficiency condition of body fluids leads to general or localized dryness and heat and an eventual inflammatory situation, while an accumulation of fluids results in a build-up of mucus and phlegm, usually due, as we have seen, to a deficiency of the Yang Root of the Kidneys[19] leading to an inability to keep fluids controlled. This will lead to such conditions as edema and other water metabolism disturbances.

MERIDIAN-ENERGETIC SYSTEMS

The meridians are the surface manifestations of the organ-energetic functional units and serve to connect the body surface with internal functioning. As such, the meridians serve as a two-way communication network, both conveying messages to the surface concerning internal malfunction (such as pain along a meridian, which signals a specific type of disturbance in the organ-energetic function associated with it), and alerting the internal functions that a surface phenomenon (such as a long-term build-up of tension and spasms) threatens to move deeper so that the bodymind's defensive energetic systems might be activated, to contain the disturbance on the surface where it is easier to combat. A *shock absorber* and *monitor of internal distress*, the meridian-energetic network is what maintains the energetic homeostasis of the bodymind. Preventing undue accumulations in one zone or unnecessary energetic waste during the performance of normal tasks in the organism, the meridians are like irrigation channels that feed and nourish, at the same time moving the flows of the bodymind to prevent stoppage. In some ways they are parallel to what we in the West call the blood vessels and the nerves, but are thought to be what propels the vessels and nerves to function—a sort of invisible web of energetic circuitry guiding the circulation of blood and the impulses to and from the nerve fibers. In brief, the meridian-energetic system is the *physics of the bodymind*, underlying the bodymind's biochemistry.

Each meridian has an internal branch (represented on the diagrams to follow by a dotted line), which is the internal energetic connection between the meridian's surface branch and the organ-energetic function of the same name (Lung, Heart, and so forth). Every meridian also possesses a surface branch (represented on the diagrams to follow by a solid line) composed of sensitive points along a particular, palpable pathway. These points are what acupuncture therapists needle, both to have a direct effect in the local area of needle insertion and to manipulate the flow of energy along the external and internal pathways of the meridian.

There are twelve regular meridians, six Yin and six Yang, each associated with an internal organ-energetic function. There are also eight extraordinary meridians, thought to develop prenatally before the development of the meridians, which constitute a fundamental network that connects meridians of the same polarity, whether Yin or Yang. In addition, there is a system of secondary vessels situated more superficially than the other meridians, which constitute the bodymind's defensive external armor.[20]

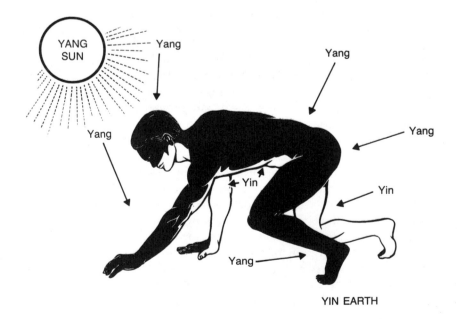

DESTINY

If you wish to receive a copy of the latest INNER TRADITIONS INTERNATIONAL catalog and to be placed on our mailing list, please send us this card.

Date _____

Name _____

Address _____

City _____ State _____ Zip _____

(Please Print)

DES

INNER TRADITIONS INTERNATIONAL, INC.

One Park Street

Rochester, VT 05767

The six Yang meridians flow along the lateral aspect of the arms and legs, the face, and the back, while the Yin meridians flow along the inner aspect of the arms and legs and the pelvic and thoracic regions. If the human body were depicted on all fours, the aspects of the body surface exposed to the sun, itself Yang, would constitute the pathways of the Yang meridians, while the aspects open to the Earth, itself Yin, would constitute the Yin meridian zones.

The surface circulation of energy through the meridians is thought to follow this order: Lung → Large Intestine → Stomach → Spleen → Heart → Small Intestine → Urinary Bladder → Kidney → Pericardium → Triple Heater → Gallbladder → Liver → . . . Lung →, accounting for the order of presentation in the table that follows on page 44.

Meridians flow in such a way that paired meridians of the same Element (e.g., Lung and Large Intestine are paired meridians of the Metal Element), as well as upper and lower branches of meridians of the same name and energetic "charge" (*Upper* and *Lower Greater Yin, Upper* and *Lower Sunlight Yang,* and so forth), are connected. This results in a multiplicity of complex connections and interrelations that, once mastered, allow the acupuncture therapist to make subtle energetic interventions to restore harmony to the bodymind's energetic flows and transformations. (See table on page 44.)

The reader may wish to mark the illustrations that follow (pages 47–66) for ready reference, as they will be referred to in Part II of this book.

In the foregoing discussion of traditional acupuncture energetics, the reader was familiarized with the ancient Chinese theory of the body as force field. This theory of energetic circulation has been submitted to a significant number of tests over the past thirty-five years in Japan and China and over the past fifteen years in the West. The results of this research indicate that the meridians are electromagnetic conductors of an as yet undetermined nature.

Physicians in the East and the West have demonstrated, through the use of various devices that measure electric current, that there is lower skin resistance and hence greater potential for electromagnetic conductivity, over at least fifty percent of the acupuncture points. While research to date concerning the electrical phenomena of the meridians and points of acupuncture have received various interpretations, results suggest that the meridians "are a kind of axis for the biological electricity of the body, or an electric circuit, a special kind of electron or electron 'bundle' which passes electromagnetic waves along a fixed course; that the electric phenomena of the skin reflect the electromagnetic field within the body,"[21] which in turn corresponds to the electromagnetic forces of nature.

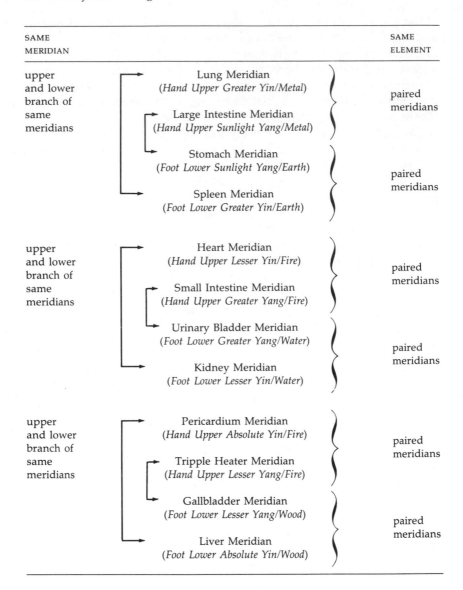

SAME MERIDIAN		SAME ELEMENT
upper and lower branch of same meridians	Lung Meridian (*Hand Upper Greater Yin/Metal*)	paired meridians
	Large Intestine Meridian (*Hand Upper Sunlight Yang/Metal*)	
	Stomach Meridian (*Foot Lower Sunlight Yang/Earth*)	paired meridians
	Spleen Meridian (*Foot Lower Greater Yin/Earth*)	
upper and lower branch of same meridians	Heart Meridian (*Hand Upper Lesser Yin/Fire*)	paired meridians
	Small Intestine Meridian (*Hand Upper Greater Yang/Fire*)	
	Urinary Bladder Meridian (*Foot Lower Greater Yang/Water*)	paired meridians
	Kidney Meridian (*Foot Lower Lesser Yin/Water*)	
upper and lower branch of same meridians	Pericardium Meridian (*Hand Upper Absolute Yin/Fire*)	paired meridians
	Tripple Heater Meridian (*Hand Upper Lesser Yang/Fire*)	
	Gallbladder Meridian (*Foot Lower Lesser Yang/Wood*)	paired meridians
	Liver Meridian (*Foot Lower Absolute Yin/Wood*)	

Most researchers also agree that the electromagnetic phenomena conducted by the meridian circuitry are mediated through the central nervous system.

Dr. Robert Becker, a pioneer in research on the electromagnetic foundations of regeneration and related healing phenomena, conducted an impressive series of experiments over a decade ago to ascertain whether, indeed, the acupuncture meridians were super-conductors of electricity. Electric current grows weaker as distance increases, owing to resistance in the transmission cable of power lines, so electrical engineers commonly build in booster amplifiers at regular intervals to maintain electric signals throughout the line. Becker hypothesized that the acupuncture points, situated at regular intervals along the meridians, were such amplifiers, hundreds of DC generators like "dark stars sending their electricity along the meridians, an interior galaxy"[22] discovered and explored over two thousand years ago by ancient Chinese physicians.

If the points were like electrical amplifiers, Becker further postulated, then the insertion of a needle into a point would contact the tissue fluid in the nearby vicinity, shorting out the pain signal. And if the integrity of healing in the bodymind is maintained, as the ancient Chinese physicians believe and Becker's theory in *The Body Electric* concurs, by a balanced circulation of this invisible electromagnetic energy, then the "various patterns of needle placement might indeed bring the circuits into harmony."[23]

Becker's research confirmed the Eastern research. Fully half of the points measured showed lesser resistance and greater electroconductivity, showing that the meridians measured served as conductors of electricity flowing into the central nervous system. Becker and his coresearchers were sufficiently impressed by their findings to conclude that the major aspects of the acupuncture-energetic system were objectively verifiable, and further research may determine the nature of the differences in potential from one point to another along a given meridian pathway. Becker concluded, on the basis of further research regarding the electromagnetic foundations of human functioning, that the anatomical structure carrying this energetic circulation was the perineural cells.[24] The use in orthopedic surgery of electrical stimulation to prompt the healing of fractured bones developed out of, and confirmed, Becker's hypothesis. Acupuncture treatment further corroborates this finding, as the stimulation by acupuncture of points above and below a healing bone seems to serve essentially the same function as electric stimulation.

It may well be that acupuncture energetics contains within its premises a first, rather complex approximation of what Becker terms the *body electric*. This energetic circuitry, this atlas of bodymind electromagnetic flow, was discovered thousands of years ago and still serves as the basis upon which millions of people are treated by acupuncture around the world today. It constitutes a bio-electric self that the new bodymind energetic paradigm of health cannot ignore.

It is our hypothesis that acupuncture energetics serves as a strong foundation upon which to explore and treat *somatic energetic reaction patterns* of the bodymind. The stimulation of meridians, by way of the acupuncture points, leads to a *resonance* with archaic, previously functional energetic pathways and serves to prod the bodymind to reactivate these pathways, leading to more appropriate responses to internal and external stress.

The acupuncture energetic concept of the bodymind can elucidate aspects of the psychosomatic question that Western psychosomatic medicine has failed to explain. As we shall see in Chapter 4, classic psychosomatics was plagued by the fact that no neurological foundations could be established for specific psychosomatic complexes. The symbolic meaning of a psychosomatic disorder could be ascertained, while the somatic component remained undefined.

While acupuncture energetics does provide answers concerning the somatic energetic nature of bodymind functioning, and while the acupuncture perspective does allow for a concept of psychic or spiritual functioning in the somatic energetic functions themselves, it is not psychologically refined enough to constitute what we in the West know as personality or ego psychology. This has led certain Western acupuncture therapists, as we shall see in the next chapter, to expand upon the acupuncture bodymind theory in order to develop an acupuncture theory of personality, and thereby modernize, from a psychosomatic perspective, this ancient bodymind-energetic model.

LUNG MERIDIAN

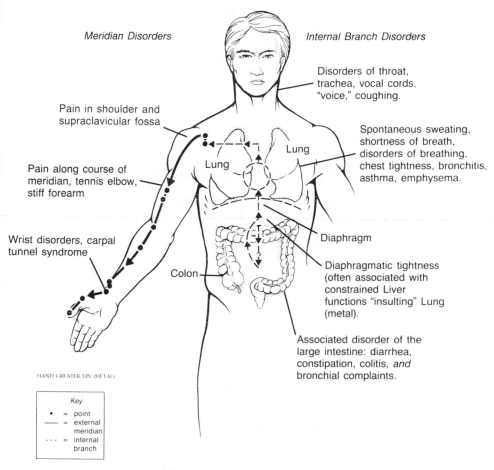

Meridian Disorders

Internal Branch Disorders

Disorders of throat, trachea, vocal cords, "voice," coughing.

Pain in shoulder and supraclavicular fossa

Spontaneous sweating, shortness of breath, disorders of breathing, chest tightness, bronchitis, asthma, emphysema.

Pain along course of meridian, tennis elbow, stiff forearm

Lung

Lung

Lung

Wrist disorders, carpal tunnel syndrome

Diaphragm

Colon

Diaphragmatic tightness (often associated with constrained Liver functions "insulting" Lung (metal).

HAND GREATER YIN (METAL)

Associated disorder of the large intestine: diarrhea, constipation, colitis, *and* bronchial complaints.

Key
• = point
—— = external meridian
- - - = internal branch

HAND GREATER YIN (METAL)

47

LARGE INTESTINE MERIDIAN

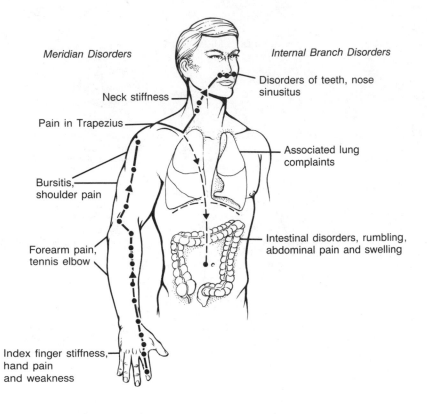

Meridian Disorders

Internal Branch Disorders

Neck stiffness

Disorders of teeth, nose sinusitus

Pain in Trapezius

Associated lung complaints

Bursitis, shoulder pain

Forearm pain, tennis elbow

Intestinal disorders, rumbling, abdominal pain and swelling

Index finger stiffness, hand pain and weakness

HAND SUNLIGHT YANG (METAL)

STOMACH MERIDIAN

Meridian Disorders

Internal Branch Disorders

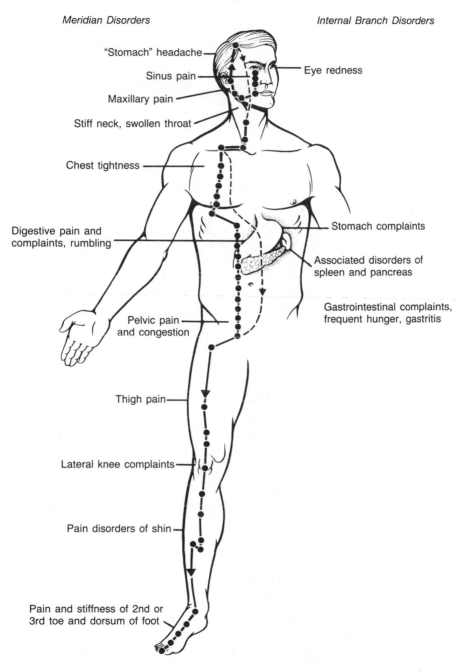

"Stomach" headache

Sinus pain

Maxillary pain

Stiff neck, swollen throat

Chest tightness

Digestive pain and complaints, rumbling

Pelvic pain and congestion

Thigh pain

Lateral knee complaints

Pain disorders of shin

Pain and stiffness of 2nd or 3rd toe and dorsum of foot

Eye redness

Stomach complaints

Associated disorders of spleen and pancreas

Gastrointestinal complaints, frequent hunger, gastritis

FOOT SUNLIGHT YANG (EARTH)

SPLEEN MERIDIAN

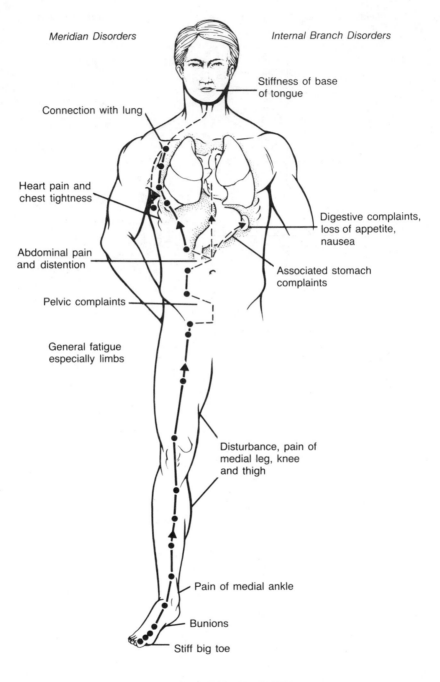

Meridian Disorders

Internal Branch Disorders

Stiffness of base of tongue

Connection with lung

Heart pain and chest tightness

Digestive complaints, loss of appetite, nausea

Abdominal pain and distention

Associated stomach complaints

Pelvic complaints

General fatigue especially limbs

Disturbance, pain of medial leg, knee and thigh

Pain of medial ankle

Bunions

Stiff big toe

FOOT GREATER YIN (EARTH)

HEART MERIDIAN

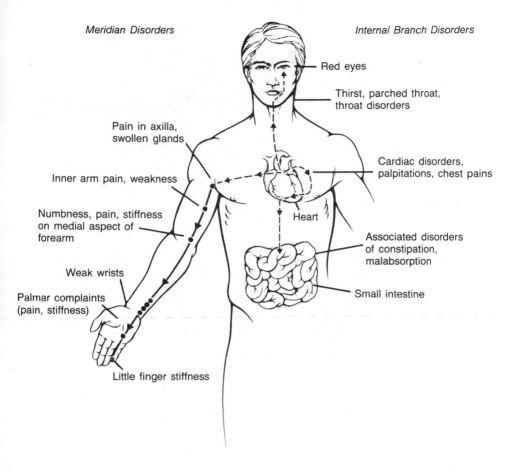

Meridian Disorders

Internal Branch Disorders

Red eyes

Thirst, parched throat, throat disorders

Pain in axilla, swollen glands

Cardiac disorders, palpitations, chest pains

Inner arm pain, weakness

Numbness, pain, stiffness on medial aspect of forearm

Heart

Associated disorders of constipation, malabsorption

Weak wrists

Small intestine

Palmar complaints (pain, stiffness)

Little finger stiffness

HAND LESSER YIN (FIRE)

SMALL INTESTINE MERIDIAN

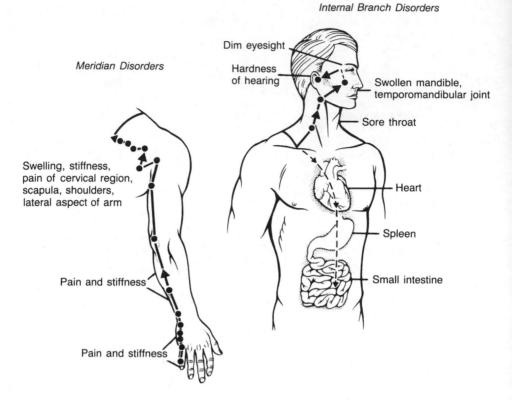

Internal Branch Disorders

Dim eyesight

Hardness of hearing

Swollen mandible, temporomandibular joint

Sore throat

Meridian Disorders

Swelling, stiffness, pain of cervical region, scapula, shoulders, lateral aspect of arm

Heart

Spleen

Small intestine

Pain and stiffness

Pain and stiffness

HAND GREATER YANG (FIRE)

BLADDER MERIDIAN

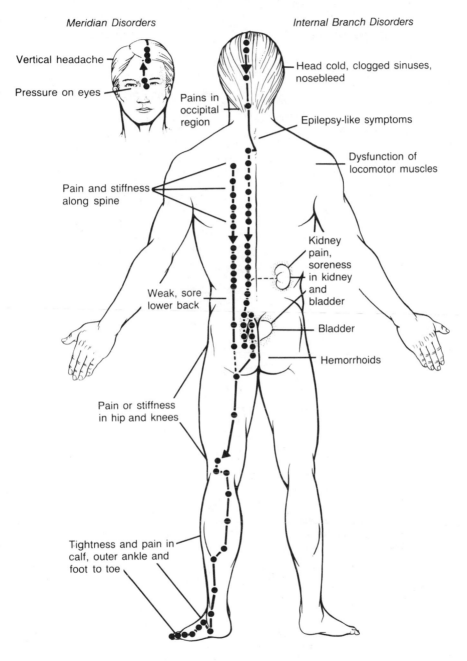

Meridian Disorders

Vertical headache

Pressure on eyes

Pains in occipital region

Pain and stiffness along spine

Weak, sore lower back

Pain or stiffness in hip and knees

Tightness and pain in calf, outer ankle and foot to toe

Internal Branch Disorders

Head cold, clogged sinuses, nosebleed

Epilepsy-like symptoms

Dysfunction of locomotor muscles

Kidney pain, soreness in kidney and bladder

Bladder

Hemorrhoids

FOOT GREATER YANG (WATER)

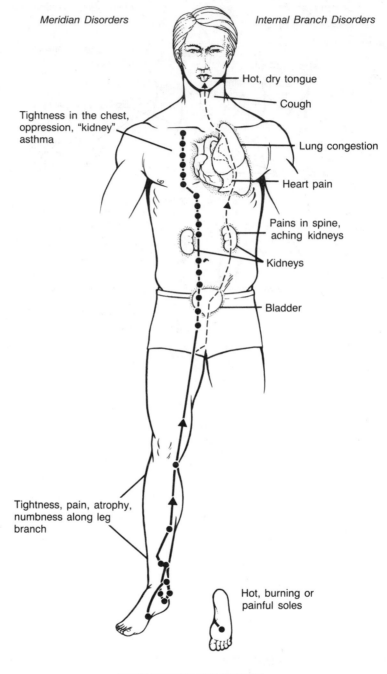

Meridian Disorders

Internal Branch Disorders

Hot, dry tongue

Cough

Tightness in the chest, oppression, "kidney" asthma

Lung congestion

Heart pain

Pains in spine, aching kidneys

Kidneys

Bladder

Tightness, pain, atrophy, numbness along leg branch

Hot, burning or painful soles

FOOT LESSER YIN (WATER)

PERICARDIUM MERIDIAN

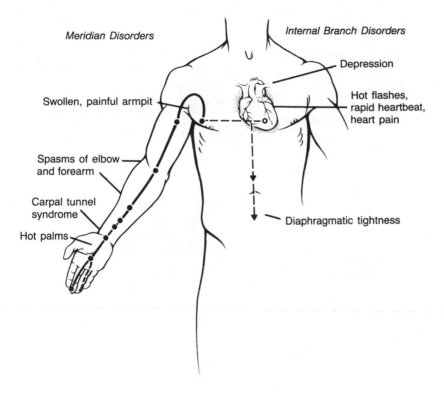

Meridian Disorders

Internal Branch Disorders

Swollen, painful armpit

Spasms of elbow and forearm

Carpal tunnel syndrome

Hot palms

Depression

Hot flashes, rapid heartbeat, heart pain

Diaphragmatic tightness

HAND ABSOLUTE YIN (FIRE)

TRIPLE WARMER MERIDIAN

Meridian Disorders   *Internal Branch Disorders*

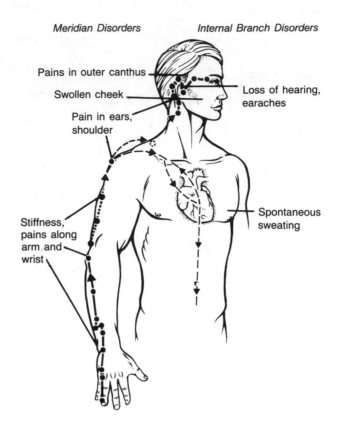

Pains in outer canthus

Swollen cheek

Pain in ears, shoulder

Loss of hearing, earaches

Stiffness, pains along arm and wrist

Spontaneous sweating

HAND LESSER YANG (FIRE)

GALLBLADDER MERIDIAN

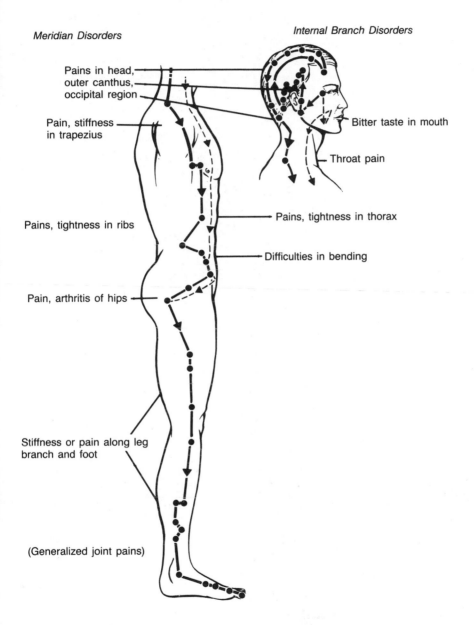

Meridian Disorders

Internal Branch Disorders

Pains in head,
outer canthus,
occipital region

Pain, stiffness
in trapezius

Pains, tightness in ribs

Pain, arthritis of hips

Stiffness or pain along leg
branch and foot

(Generalized joint pains)

Bitter taste in mouth

Throat pain

Pains, tightness in thorax

Difficulties in bending

FOOT LESSER YANG (WOOD)

LIVER MERIDIAN

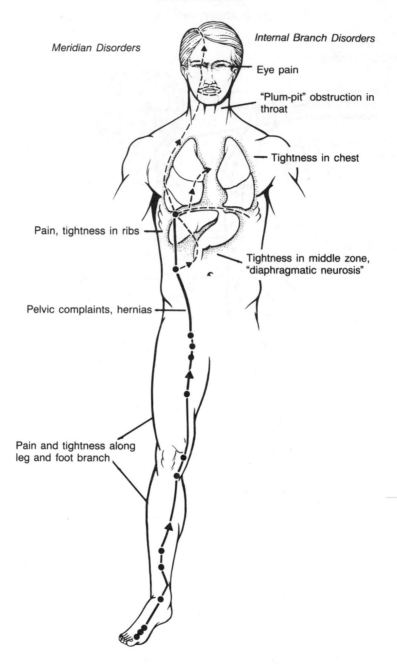

Meridian Disorders

Internal Branch Disorders

Eye pain

"Plum-pit" obstruction in throat

Tightness in chest

Pain, tightness in ribs

Tightness in middle zone, "diaphragmatic neurosis"

Pelvic complaints, hernias

Pain and tightness along leg and foot branch

FOOT ABSOLUTE YIN (WOOD)

THE EIGHT EXTRA VESSELS

CONCEPTION VESSEL (YIN)

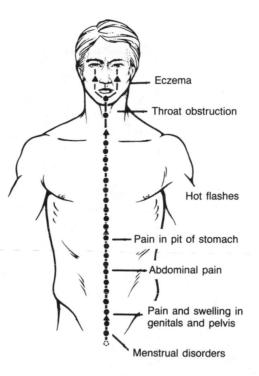

GOVERNING VESSEL (YANG)

Vertical headache

Eye pains

Stiff neck

Spasms, pain in spine,
epileptic-like symptoms,
urinary incontinence,
impotence or sterility

Hemorrhoids, hernias

THRUSTING VESSEL (YIN)

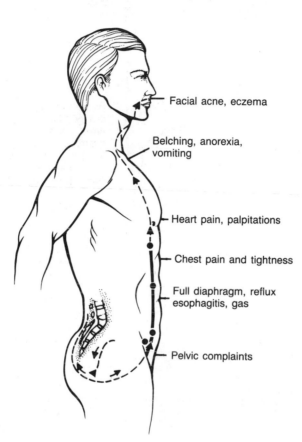

Facial acne, eczema

Belching, anorexia, vomiting

Heart pain, palpitations

Chest pain and tightness

Full diaphragm, reflux esophagitis, gas

Pelvic complaints

BELT CHANNEL (YANG)

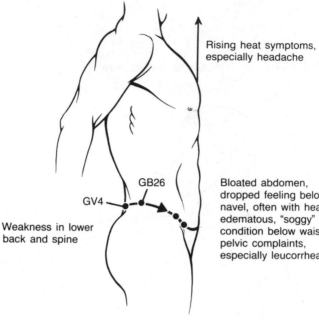

Rising heat symptoms, especially headache

GB26

GV4

Weakness in lower back and spine

Bloated abdomen, dropped feeling below navel, often with heavy, edematous, "soggy" condition below waist, pelvic complaints, especially leucorrhea

YIN HEEL VESSEL (YIN)

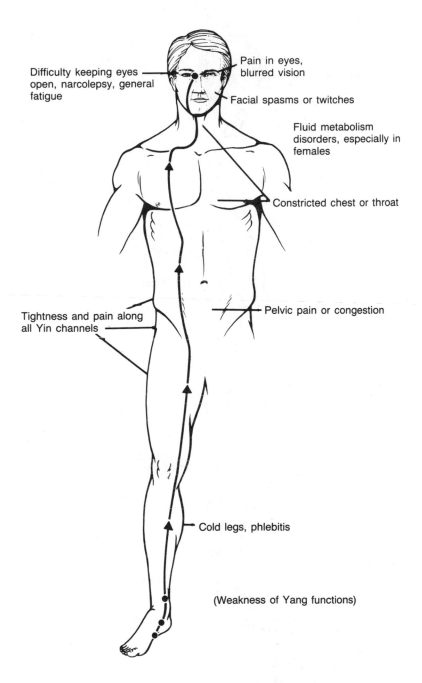

Difficulty keeping eyes open, narcolepsy, general fatigue

Pain in eyes, blurred vision

Facial spasms or twitches

Fluid metabolism disorders, especially in females

Constricted chest or throat

Pelvic pain or congestion

Tightness and pain along all Yin channels

Cold legs, phlebitis

(Weakness of Yang functions)

YANG HEEL VESSEL (YANG)

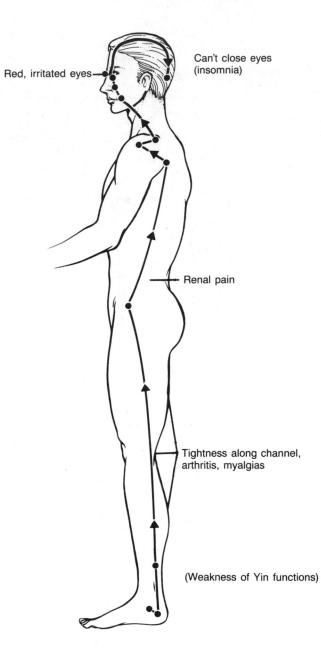

Red, irritated eyes

Can't close eyes
(insomnia)

Renal pain

Tightness along channel,
arthritis, myalgias

(Weakness of Yin functions)

YIN REGULATING VESSEL (YIN)

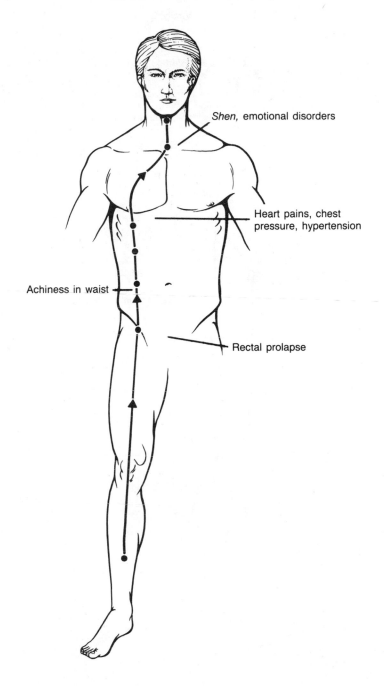

Shen, emotional disorders

Heart pains, chest pressure, hypertension

Achiness in waist

Rectal prolapse

YANG REGULATING VESSEL (YANG)

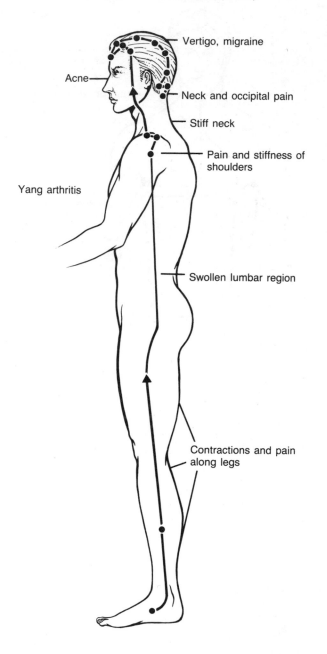

Vertigo, migraine

Acne

Neck and occipital pain

Stiff neck

Pain and stiffness of shoulders

Yang arthritis

Swollen lumbar region

Contractions and pain along legs

CHAPTER SUMMARY

Philosophical Bases of Acupuncture Energetics

YinYang and the *Five Phases* constitute the philosophical bases or organizing metaphors of traditional Chinese medicine.

All living things are composed of two complementary forces, which are termed Yin and Yang. Everything possesses both a Yin and a Yang aspect in such a way that Yin may transform at its apogee into Yang and vice versa, constituting a theory of relativity appropriate to the study of human beings.

For clinical purposes, a patient's signs and symptoms may be categorized as Yin or Yang; the framework is customarily expanded into the *Eight Guiding Criteria* or *Eight Principal Patterns*. In addition to *Yin* and *Yang*, these criteria include *Interior* and *Exterior*, which refers both to the location of a disorder and to the direction from or toward which it develops; *Deficiency* and *Excess*, which refers to the relative quantity of force at work; and *Cold* and *Hot*, which refers to the quality of an imbalance.

The *Five Phases* or *Five Elements* is the second organizing metaphor of acupuncture energetics. It postulates specific connections between the organ-energetic functions of the bodymind, and a series of detailed correspondences that allow the acupuncture therapist to observe the energetic traces left in the bodymind and to decipher them by fitting them into a pattern of energetic disharmony specific to the individual.

Points may be selected for treatment based on either the YinYang or the Five Phase theory, or a combination of both perspectives, to restore energetic balance in a disturbed function or zone of the bodymind.

The *generation* and *control cycles* of the Five Phase theory depict the normal energetic physiological relationships of the organ-functional units, and the *destruction* and *violation* cycles explain the dynamics of pathological reaction patterns.

Energetic-Functional Spheres

When organs are named in traditional Chinese medicine they refer to energetic-functional units rather than, as in Western medicine, to the somatic structures involved. In the acupuncture-energetic model, there are twelve major organ-energetic functional units, six Yin and six Yang. The Yin and Yang organ functions work in pairs with one Yin and one Yang function interconnected. Additionally, each pair is associated with one of the Five Phases or Elements.

Energetically, each organ function has a Yin (storing and nourishing) as well as a Yang (active and protective) aspect, stemming from the Yin and Yang Root of the Kidneys, which store the bodymind's energetic potential *(ancestral energy)*. A relative tendency toward deficiency of either the Yin or Yang Root is usually present in an individual and affects the major corresponding Yin or Yang functions. This aids the therapist in predicting the nature of the phenomenological development of an individual's energetic imbalances, along a "becoming hot" or a "becoming cold" course.

Manifestations of Energy

Acupuncture-energetic theory postulates a division of the bodymind into several fundamental substances: Qi (Energy), Blood, Body Fluids, Ancestral Energy, and Spirit (Shen).

Meridian Energetics

The meridians are the surface manifestations of the organ-energetic functional units and connect the surface of the body with internal functioning; so the meridians may be seen as shock absorbers and monitors of internal function. Modern research depicts the meridians of acupuncture as superconductors of electromagnetic energy, so that treatment by acupuncture therapy can be understood as a means of regulating the functions of the body electric to restore normalcy to the bio-electric self.

While the acupuncture-energetic conception of the bodymind provides answers to many aspects of the psychosomatic question as raised in the West, concerning somatic energetic functioning, Western practitioners must expand upon the psychoenergetic aspects of acupuncture to develop a bodymind-energetic theory adequate to the new paradigm of health that is emerging.

NOTES

1. Claude Larre, Jean Schatz, Elizabeth Rochat de la Vallée, *Survey of Traditional Chinese Medicine* (translated by Sarah Elizabeth Stang). Columbia, Maryland, Traditional Acupuncture Foundation, 1986, p. 59.
2. Ibid, pp. 19–21.
3. Ted J. Kaptchuk, *The Web That Has No Weaver*. New York, Congdon & Weed, 1983, pp. 7–15.
4. Ibid, pp. 178–179.
5. Ibid, pp. 181–182.
6. Ibid, p. 182.
7. Ibid, p. 182.

8. Ibid, pp. 182–183. Cf. *The Web that Has No Weaver*, pp. 181–200, for a highly readable discussion of these eight principal patterns.

9. For a discussion of the way the Five Elements and Eight Principles combine, see Mark D. Seem, *Acupuncture Energetics*. New York, Thorsons Publishers, Inc., 1986.

10. The reader will be interested to know that there is a Fire, Earth, Metal, Water, and Wood point for each organ function, located on the corresponding meridians between the toes and knees, or fingers and elbows, so that Five Element treatment has a corporeal reality in the points themselves.

11. It should be noted that while modern China has forsaken the Five Phase approach, this approach is still very much utilized in constitutional Korean acupuncture, in many Japanese traditions, and throughout Europe and the United States.

12. *The Web That Has No Weaver*, pp. 51–52. Cf. also Porkert, *Theoretical Foundations of Chinese Medicine*, Chapter 3, pp. 107–166; and Capra, *The Turning Point*, pp. 313–314.

13. An important effort in this direction is the detailed work of Dr. Yves Requena, in *Terrains and Pathology in Acupuncture*, Brookline, Mass., Paradigm Publications, 1986, which tends, unfortunately, to strict parallels that bear the weight of a Western medical view.

14. Especially Kaptchuk, *The Web That Has No Weaver*; Porkert, *Theoretical Foundations of Traditional Chinese Medicine*; and Seem, *Acupuncture Energetics*.

15. For more details see *Acupuncture Energetics* by Mark D. Seem.

16. Kaptchuk, *The Web That Has No Weaver*, p. 36.

17. Ibid, pp. 34–46 and 201–204 for a detailed discussion of these energetic substances and their disturbances.

18. We shall look at this spiritual, personalized concept of organ energetic functions in Chapter 3.

19. In conditions of a deficiency of the Yang Root of the Kidneys, the Yang function of transportation and transformation of foods and fluids in the Spleen will also be weakened.

20. These secondary meridians, namely the tendino-muscular, divergent, longitudinal, and tranverse luo vessels, are beyond the confines of this brief introduction. For further details, see Royston Low, *The Secondary Vessels of Acupuncture*. London, Thorsons Publishing Group, 1984.

21. One of the difficulties in such research lies in the interference caused by the electrical detection devices themselves. The reader is referred to *Acupuncture: A Comprehensive Text*, by the Shanghai College of Traditional Chinese Medicine, translated with commentary by John O'Connor and Dan Bensky. Chicago, Eastland Press, 1981, pp. 105–111.

22. Robert O. Becker, M.D., and Gary Selden, *The Body Electric, Electromagnetism and the Foundations of Life*. New York, William Morrow & Company, 1985, pp. 234–235.

23. Ibid, p. 235.

24. The reader is referred to the entirety of Becker's research summarized in *The Body Electric*, pp. 236–237 regarding acupuncture.

3

Acupuncture Personality Theories and Predisposition to Disease

> The Chinese system is holistic only in theory . . . . There is no psychotherapy and there is no attempt to give patients advice on how they could change their life situation.[1]
>
> Fritjof Capra

THE PSYCHOLOGICAL SUBJECT

As we saw in Chapter 2, the Chinese medical model takes the psychological life of the individual into account only to the extent that correspondences exist between each of the Five Phases and an emotional and behavioral disposition. For example, the Wood phase (Liver and Gallbladder organ-energetic functions) is associated with a tendency toward an angry disposition and behavioral disturbances in planning and decision making. While a Chinese traditional doctor may notice these psychological traits and use them as additional data in his diagnosis, he will neither deal with the psychological issues per se, counsel the patient on ways to change behavior nor offer interpretations of the psychological meaning of the complaint.

This should not be surprising, for the Confucian concept of the individual, which has dominated Chinese society for centuries and influenced the development of traditional Chinese medicine, consists not of a psychological Self but rather of the Self actively involved with community (the family, the province, the state, and the world). Self-cultivation and self-awareness, central to the Confucian formulation of individual existence, were perceived as practices of spiritual development that related the individual to his community, including family heritage.[2]

The Self in ancient Chinese culture was therefore essentially a social Self. Rather than a *psychology of the individual*, then, the Chinese developed a *sociology of the Self*. Behavioral problems that we in the West understand as psychological problems of personality development would be viewed in China as essentially social problems of adaptation and adjustment. Thus, an individual whose behavior deviates from the normal would not be referred to a medical or psychological specialist but to the communal group, which would comprehend the problem on a social, rather than a medical or psychotherapeutic, level.[3]

This is in marked contrast to the Western Self, which is perceived as an isolated, alienated being. The Western Self, from the end of the nineteenth century on, has been depicted as a Self divorced from the spiritual realm and alienated from fellow human beings.[4] Such a view paralleled the development of modern psychology and psychiatry, which defined this alienated Self as a subject for psychological scrutiny. The psychological subject (ego) central to the practice of psychology, psychiatry, and psychotherapy in the West is virtually nonexistent in China. There is no psychotherapy in China, nor have Western psychological concepts been adopted, even though there is a widespread adoption, and even preeminence, of the Western medical model.

For instance, a patient in China who experiences what we in the West call "depression" will tend to somatize the experience (experience it within the body) rather than experience it psychologically. Consulting a traditional physician or acupuncture therapist, the patient will focus on specific bodily dysfunctions such as tightness in the chest or a closed feeling in the throat. The practitioner will prescribe an acupuncture treatment or a formula of herbs to restore smooth functioning in the constricted zones of the body. Relief of the symptoms will enable the patient to breath more easily and, to the extent that tightness in the chest or throat is a concomitant of depression, may perhaps facilitate "psychic breathing" as well. This will occur as a side effect of therapy rather than as a stated objective. Cultural dictates are such that even a discreet inquiry on the part of the practitioner into the life situation of the patient is virtually impossible.[5] Thus, the opportunity for the Chinese patient to make an association between the bodily felt experience of constriction and the constraints imposed by social circumstances is lacking.

In contrast, Western practitioners commonly find that their patients have already made associations between their physical problems and their psychological state of mind. This is not to imply that one or the other experience and concept of the Self is superior or preferable to the other. Cultural differences in how an individual experiences self-hood cannot be ignored nor can one experience be used to criticize another.[6] This is why we must be very careful, in adopting a Chinese acupuncture-energetic model in the West, to reconstruct this model in a way that takes account of our modes of psychological being-in-the-world. For better or worse, the Western individual is a psychological being, and this aspect of the patient must be taken into account by any acupuncture therapist wishing to do more than purely symptomatic acupuncture.[7]

Acupuncture therapy, while unblocking an energetic zone, simultaneously frees up the psyche trapped in that zone, and if attention is not paid to the underlying psychological issues in the patient's life experience, a new energetic zone will soon become disturbed. This results in constantly shifting or wandering symptoms, a kind of energetic hysteria due to the practitioner's inability or unwillingness to focus on the soul as well as the body. It has been a shared experience of some acupuncture therapists in the West that subsequent to mastering the use of acupuncture to treat *somatic energetic* disturbances (energetic treatment from the side of the body), they begin moving toward a practice that includes treatment of *psychoenergetic* imbalances as well (energetic treatment from the side of the psyche).[8] The necessity for treating at the psychological and spiritual levels is evident in the practice of American acupuncture conceived as a bodymind-energetic therapy. As Eric Stephens, an American acupuncturist, states of his own development, one becomes increasingly more aware "of the emotional, mental and spiritual components—they become impossible to ignore."[9] A spontaneous movement is occurring in some areas of American acupuncture toward a bodymind-energetic approach to acupuncture therapy. This approach is not identical to Chinese acupuncture, and is as influenced by English and French practices as it is by the Oriental approaches. In focusing on two European approaches to acupuncture that have attempted to expand upon the psychological side of acupuncture by constructing what might be termed acupuncture personality theories, we wish to situate these experiences with respect to this country, where acupuncture therapists must come to grips with the bodymind question. In fact, experiences such as Stephens's are reflective of an unprecedented integration of different traditions of acupuncture with a Western understanding of psychology. As he concludes, they point to "the synthesis of the Oriental tradition with psychology and other humanistic therapies, and [to] the focus on treating persons in the full context of their lives—at the emotional, mental and spiritual levels, as well as the physical."[10]

ACUPUNCTURE PERSONALITY THEORY

There are two basic ways in which the transformation of acupuncture therapy, to meet the needs of a modern Western public besieged by emotional, psychological, and spiritual concerns as well as by physical complaints, might be realized.

One is to expand upon those aspects of traditional acupuncture theory and practice that emphasize the relation between mind and body and the equal importance of the physical and the spiritual realms, extracting and enriching the psychological elements contained in the classic texts. This would provide us with a means, from within the acupuncture perspective, for speaking about the personality, and not only the energetic imbalances, of our clients, resulting in a kind of *acupuncture personality theory*. Two examples of such acupuncture personality theories, one from France and one from England, will be discussed in the following pages.

A second way in which acupuncture therapy might be refined for use in the West would be to juxtapose acupuncture energetics and appropriate psychological models to develop an expanded concept of bodymind interaction, and a collaborative approach among acupuncturists, somatic therapists, and psychotherapists. This possibility will be explored in Chapters 4–10. Either approach would lead to a bodymind-energetic approach with great potential for contributing to the newly emerging paradigm of health and health care.

Personality and Typing

Before proceeding with a discussion of acupuncture personality theories, a clarification of what is generally meant by *personality* is in order.

Western psychology tends to use the term "personality" to denote the constellation or pattern of an individual's ways of behaving, thinking, and feeling. This personality pattern is the result of a complex combination of inherited and acquired physiological and social forces, with proponents who emphasize physiological as opposed to social forces, or inherited as opposed to acquired tendencies (and the reverse) as the key in dictating the nature of a given personality.[11]

In attempting to study the psychological differences between one personality and another, the issue of classifying people into personality types arises. Historically, the attempt to define personality traits or types has been prominent: from Hippocrates' classification of people into four basic "temperaments" (sanguine, melancholic, choleric, and phlegmatic) according to the dominance of body "humors" (respectively, red blood, black bile, yellow bile, and phlegm); to Carl Jung's classification, based on the directionality of energy toward the outside world ("extroversion") or toward the internal ("introversion"); to W. H. Sheldon's constitutional theory based on three somatotypes (the round, soft, "endomorphic" body type; the strong, muscular, "mesomorphic" body type; and the flat-chested, fragile, "ectomorphic" body type, each of which exhibits a different personality pattern).[12]

Debates concerning the crucial factors in personality development generally arise between trait theorists who believe that certain consistent traits define personality, and situationists who argue that personality patterns are largely determined by the characteristics of a given situation rather than by the traits of the individual. A useful compromise proposed by some is a perspective that emphasizes the specific *interaction* between a given individual and a specific situation.

Reaction Patterns, Not Character Traits

An interesting example of the interactionist position, the position we shall adopt to situate the following discussion of acupuncture personality theories, is implicit in Wilhelm Reich's theory of "character armoring."

In Reich's theory, the personality or "character" is defined by the chronic *mode of reaction* of the individual on the one hand, and the specific *types of situations,* on the other, in which the individual is subjected to recurrent conflicts between internal needs and desires and the inhibition of these desires by an anxiety-producing modern world. As Reich states it, "it is as if the affective personality armored itself, as if the hard shell it develops were intended to deflect and weaken the blows of the outer world as well as the clamoring of internal needs."[13] Seeing the psyche and the soma as a functional unit, Reich stressed that the armoring, while in the body's surface musculature, is psychoenergetic in nature. The "muscular rigidity and the psychic rigidity are a unit, the sign of a disturbance of the vegetative motility of the biological system as a whole."[14]

Reich stresses further that this character armoring requires energy, and is sustained by the psychic and somatic energies of the bodymind, resulting in a lessened ability for the bodymind to function smoothly and in harmony with its internal and external environments. The goal of Reich's character analysis was to break down this armor, which he viewed as a dysfunctional process that absorbed and consumed inhibited energy in the bodymind. Once this armor was broken down, Reich postulated, energy that was originally required to sustain the armoring reaction pattern could be put to more creative use.

This view of psychological defense mechanisms, as somatic reaction patterns (character armoring) fueled by psychological and physical energies, defines the bodymind as a *psychosomatic energetic unit.*

The shift of emphasis, away from an individual's personal traits and toward his or her *patterns of reaction* in given conflict situations, enables us to avoid developing fixed character typologies. While it is natural, in discussing personality, to classify people's traits and arrive at types (a *friendly* person, an *efficient* worker, an *empathic* therapist, and so on), the danger in developing an acupuncture personality typology is that it shifts the acupuncture therapist's focus away from the dynamics of the bodymind to some rather rigid fixed classificatory system.

The phenomenological perspective on acupuncture energetics developed in Chapter 2 focuses less on patterns of disharmony or imbalances (still a pathologizing perspective, inherent in the modern development of traditional Chinese medicine and acupuncture, that focuses on illness rather than well-being) and more on *patterns of reaction.* In speaking of reaction patterns, whether psychic or somatic, one is immediately immersed in the complex web of interactions that connect any given person's ways of coping at a given time with specific circumstances and a multiplicity of internal and external factors. To speak of a reaction pattern specific to an individual with a deficiency in the Fire Element, or with an imbalance in the Heart Official, with respect to a specific situation, or to speak of a reaction pattern that brings into play the entire functional energetic unit of the Gallbladder and Triple Heater systems, is altogether different from speaking of a Fire "Type" or a Gallbladder and Triple Heater (Lesser Yang) "Temperament."

The Danger of Typing

To speak of the personality pattern of an individual as that individual's energy and way of expending it, emotional tone, attitudes, interests, values, and other characteristics, easily leads to a perspective that reduces the person to a combination of traits. By and large, character typologies have fallen into disrepute precisely because they are prone to facile application. Advocates of any theory of types face the danger of becoming so absorbed in correctly assessing a person's "type" that they lose sight of a bodymind energetic therapist's essential task: to meet a client within that client's own experience of being-in-the-world and to support the client's efforts to heal himself or herself and become more whole.

Acupuncture therapists frequently speak, for example, of a Liver "Type" or a Water "Type," which really is a way of speaking about the specific reaction patterns of a person experiencing disturbances in Liver organ-energetic functioning or within the Water Element and its complex energetic functions. Such utterances reflect the need to classify data, and if used properly, such personal, pragmatic personality typing is simply the therapist's way of grasping some of the central issues in the client and developing some parameters from which to begin an exploration *with* and *for* that person.

The real danger in typing is that it can serve as a shield behind which the therapist hides, a device for labeling people and their problems into neat categories. Such a labeling process protects the therapist from the often experienced anxiety of not knowing what is going on in the patient's bodymind, and obliterates any possibility for open communication between therapist and client (a situation that has arisen in the encounter between the medical doctor and the patient).[15] The phenomenological, experiential nature of the bodymind-energetic approach that we are advocating obviates any possibility for adopting the doctor–patient relationship as the model for the therapeutic relationship.

This long prelude to a discussion of acupuncture personality theories is meant to serve as a caution against adopting mechanistic typing procedures to the detriment of the dynamic nature of acupuncture energetics. While the psychological side of acupuncture must be expanded, it must be done in a way consistent with the bodymind energetic complexity inherent in the acupuncture approach.

Two Acupuncture Personality Theories

Two acupuncture personality theories – the "Twelve Officials and Five Elements" of Professor J. R. Worsley and the "Five Acupuncture Constitutions and Eight Temperaments" of Dr. Yves Requena[16] – have been chosen to illustrate ways in which, beginning with Chinese medical traditions, Western practitioners have attempted to expand upon the psychological side of acupuncture theory to establish a concept of personality.

PATTERNS OF AWARENESS

Starting from something akin to a phenomenological, experiential point of view, J. R. Worsley retrieved the traditional concept of the Five Elements of acupuncture, thus enabling one to speak not only of the material substance of Fire, for instance, and all that is associated with it *in nature* (heat, fast activity, the Sun) but also of the Fire within human beings, *Human Fire* (being warm and giving warmth, emotionally and spiritually).[17] Starting from this perspective, Worsley adopted an anthropomorphic, humanized reading of the organ-energetic functions associated with each Element, resulting in the twelve personality patterns or *Twelve Officials*. While these officials are mentioned very briefly in the *Yellow Emperor's Classic of Internal Medicine* (Chapter 8), Worsley expanded upon the brief descriptions in the classics to arrive at an approach that could help Western patients begin not only to feel a part of Nature, but also to become aware of their own inner experience of the material and energetic nature of the universe. One person's dreams, and entire way of relating to the world and to other people, may be infused with references to Water and Fire, while the other Elements may be lacking. Such a person experiences the inner world as a dynamic interplay of Water and Fire, fluidity and activity, cooling and warming functions, the sea and the sun. Such observations of an inner experience of the elements of nature in human beings have been verified by phenomenological psychologists and philosophers—especially Ludwig Binswanger, a psychiatrist and one of the first Swiss followers of Freud, who later developed his own approach, Existential Analysis *(Daseinanalyse)*, and Gaston Bachelard, a French phenomenological philosopher.[18] These authors do not view references to the elements as mere metaphors of reality, but, exactly as in Worsley's Five Element concept, as "actually appearing forms and configurations of existence."[19] Phenomenological psychiatrists frequently observed a disproportion in a patient's inner experience of the elements. Regarding the case of a schizophrenic depressive patient, Minkowski, a Parisian psychiatrist and phenomenologist, noted that his inner worlds make "no mention of air, water or fire . . . but there are many references to metallic and earthly substances (materiality)."[20]

Like the phenomenologists, Worsley advocates a careful investigation of a person's inner universe to ascertain the relative dominance of some elements over others, as a first phase in reconstructing the person's inner worlds, so as to be able to effect energetic changes resulting in the more normal distribution of the Five Elements within the person's bodymind.

Once the basic imbalances in one or more Elements have been unveiled, Worsley moves on to explore which energetic functions and aspects of the individual's personality are disturbed by developing a communication with the corresponding "Officials." This anthropomorphized view of the twelve organ-energetic functions (Heart, Small Intestine, and so forth) serves as a personality theory that aids those working from the Five Element acupuncture approach to relate to an individual not only on the basis of energetic imbalances but also, more deeply, with respect to that person's inner experiences of "body-mind-spirit."

While Worsley's approach has been criticized as a distortion of traditional Chinese medical concepts, or as being based on outdated "metaphysical" constructs,[21] this decidedly Western perspective is an excellent example of an expansion of acupuncture energetics to meet the needs of modern patients, who have lost touch with their "inner worlds." Furthermore, the American extension of Worsley's Five Element school headed by Dianne Connelly and Robert Duggan,[22] who were both active in the human potential movement before turning to the study of acupuncture, represents an approach to acupuncture therapy that moves away from the modern, traditional Chinese medical model of doctor/patient/disease to a phenomenological model more in tune with the spirit of the early Taoist healing traditions of guide/explorer/experience. In this view, which might be seen as a *human potential acupuncture* perspective, diseases and symptoms are only a part of the larger picture, and the relationship of healing is one of experience and exploration of the patient's inner worlds.[23] While speaking of a person's imbalance in Fire or in the Heart Official, these practitioners focus less on the disturbance and more on *the state of health that could be achieved* if these imbalances were rectified. Rather than adopt an objective, inductive medico-scientific view of the individual's personality patterns that reduces the complex individual to a pattern of behavior or set of traits or specific "character type," these acupuncture therapists will work from a more subjective, empirical phenomenological-humanistic perspective. This perspective is much like Jung's in that the personality pattern of the individual is seen as composed of specific *patterns of awareness*[24] that must be grasped from the point of view of the person's own reality, rather than in terms of some preconceived category or concept of the therapist. The actual energetic imbalances of the individual, along with his or her awareness of these imbalances and the potential for becoming more whole and healthy, are the focus of this acupuncture approach. They fit exactly the definition of the phenomenological empirical approach, as defined by Binswanger. In such an approach, the empirical knowledge derived from the patient's own phenomenological experience is taken as the data upon which to do scientific analysis and therapeutic work. "In phenomenological experience, the discursive taking apart of natural objects into characteristics or qualities and their inductive elaboration into types, concepts, judgements, conclusions, and theories is replaced by giving expression to the content of what is purely phenomenally given."[25] Rather than making deductions about this world, therapists working from such an orientation let it speak for itself, as it is.

In like fashion, practitioners of this tradition of Five Element acupuncture do not seek to reduce people to their symptoms or diseases, but rather engage in an exploration of their clients' inner realms and gain access to stored, untapped potential, to help them become more whole in "body, mind and spirit."[26] Unfortunately, these practitioners often fail to appreciate the Yin Yang energetic nature of symptoms that would lead to proper treatment of specific disorders and complaints.

ACUPUNCTURE CHARACTER TYPING

Beginning with the work of Dr. Menetrier on trace elements and a theory of five diatheses (predispositions to disease), which he likens to the Five Elements in acupuncture, as well as the work of Dr. Gaston Berger, a French physician and pioneer in the field of biotypology (similar to the somatopsychology of Sheldon mentioned earlier) and the latter's theory of eight temperaments, Dr. Yves Requena developed an acupuncture personality theory synthesizing these typologies and what he views as a rudimentary typological system in the ancient Chinese medical texts.[27]

Requena based his work on the French characterological school of Le Senne and Berger, which delineates eight character types based on the interrelationship of three personality factors (emotivity, activity, and primary or secondary resonance), and principles from the morphopsychological school of Corman, a physiognomist. He developed correlations with the six great meridians (Greater Yin, Sunlight Yang, Lesser Yin, Greater Yang, Absolute Yin, Lesser Yang). Since each great meridian, as we saw in Chapter 2, is composed of two Elements (Greater Yin is composed of *Earth*-Spleen and *Metal*-Lung, for example), he views the six meridians as a means of building upon the five diatheses of Menetrier to develop a more detailed concept of temperament than Berger's. In this fashion, Requena claims to have solved several problems of the characterological approach, most notably its inability to pinpoint with precision the temperamental predispositions to specific diseases. The energetic perspective of acupuncture, with its multiplicity of complex correlations connecting physiological and psychological functions that remain separate in Western physiology, provides a missing link to infuse the characterological approach with new life.

An immediate difficulty with this highly ambitious enterprise is that it postulates correlations between traits attributed to each of the six energetic systems, developed only fleetingly in one chapter of the *Yellow Emperor's Classic*, and a highly developed classification system in French characterological and morphological psychology. The underlying assumption, never addressed by Requena, is that characterological and morphological traits are universal, so that one might combine traits observed by the Chinese two thousand years ago with those attributed to specific character types in modern French bio-typology. Such an ethnocentric perspective is problematic in and of itself, and is a difficulty in all attempts to develop a universal taxonomy of personality types. More troublesome is that the sketches given by the ancient Chinese observers have never been developed into a theory of types, but rather serve as broad indicators with which to begin an investigation of a person's energetic imbalances.

Worsley expands upon the twelve Officials of acupuncture in the spirit of the ancient Chinese authors, never reducing these Officials to strict traits or character types. Requena, on the other hand, combines the broad acupuncture traits with the highly specific typologies of Berger and Menetrier, forcing what is really only a glimpse of a typology in acupuncture into a decidedly rigid typological mold.[28]

By definition, a phenomenological approach focuses on being with the individual in the moment. It does not seek to reduce the patient's worlds to preconceived categories. Thus, character typing fits poorly within a phenomenological framework unless the typing is consistently relativized and downplayed. From a bodymind-energetic approach, Requena's typology does offer a new perspective on bodymind interractions, infused with the acupuncture-energetic concepts. Here we shall review in chart form the relationship between the character types of French bio-typology utilized by Requena and the six energetic "morphologies" of acupuncture. The reader is referred to Requena's texts for a detailed discussion.

EIGHT CHARACTER TYPOLOGIES AND ACUPUNCTURE

Wood-Fire	Lesser Yang	=	Choleric type	=	Emotive, Active, Primary[29]
	Absolute Yin	=	Nervous type	=	Emotive, Non-active, primary
Water-Fire	Greater Yang	=	Passionate type	=	Emotive, Active, Secondary
	Lesser Yin	=	Sentimental type	=	Emotive, Non-Active, Secondary
Earth[30]	Sunlight Yang	=	Sanguine type	=	Non-Emotive, Active, Primary
Earth[30]	Greater Yin	=	Amorphous type	=	Non-Emotive, Non-Active, Primary
Metal[30]	Sunlight Yang	=	Phlegmatic type	=	Non-Emotive, Active, Secondary
Metal[30]	Greater Yin	=	Apathetic type	=	Non-Emotive, Non-Active, Secondary

[29]The "emotive" is quick to become excited; the "non-emotive," slow; the "active" readily acts on impulses; the "non-active" delays action; the "primary" reacts in and to the present; the "secondary" reacts in and to the past, as if predetermined by it. The reader will note that "active" is equivalent to *yang*, and "non-active" to *yin*, and that the emotive types are those within the Fire element in Requena's formulation.

[30]The reader will note that in order to make the eight temperaments of Berger correlate with the six "energetic types" of acupuncture, Requena divided the Earth-Metal Types (SUNLIGHT YANG and GREATER YIN), into the EARTH and the METAL types within these larger categories. This is another example of a kind of *forcing* to make correlations fit. Another example is when Requena "reconstitutes" Absolute Yin and Yang Ming "types," not given in the Chinese classics.

The correlation between bio-typological data from the French schools and admittedly scanty references to personality traits in the *Yellow Emperor's Classic* (in which, incidentally, there is no mention of the Greater Yin or Sunlight Yang "personality traits" and description of traits for the Greater Yin poses tremendous difficulty when it is compared with the corresponding French character types[31]) seems at many points arbitrary and contradictory to the original Chinese medical intention of seizing an individual in his or her uniqueness, in the present moment, rather than assigning that individual to a class or category.

Nevertheless, Requena's approach is extremely useful to the acupuncture therapist, as it leads to focusing on the six energetic relationships and aids in developing a detailed study of which disorders and imbalances affect each of the six meridian units (Greater Yang, etc.).

As we saw earlier, the interactionist point of view does not refer to strict character types or traits but focuses on the complex interrelations between a multiplicity of factors in the situation at hand (and the factors that lead up to it), and the personality factors that bear on the individual's reactions to the situation. From this interactionist perspective, it is more judicious to speak of reaction patterns than patterns of types. If we take this view regarding Requena's work, and understand his description of the Eight Temperaments as modes of reactivity, we might refer to these eight "modes" as *somatic energetic zones*, with characteristic somatic energetic reaction patterns for each zone. In this reformulation, the emphasis is on reaction patterns already observed by the ancient Chinese authors and practitioners, and there is no need to adhere to the correlations with the French biotypologies. This in no way detracts from the importance or novelty of Requena's approach. Viewed from this perspective, his categorization of the most common Western medical diseases and disorders in terms of somatic energetic zones and their specific modes of reactivity is of use not only to acupuncture therapists but to all bodymind-energetic therapists who wish to understand the complex ways in which psyche and soma interrelate in a given disorder. His approach also sharpens the focus on energetic units (Lesser Yang, and so on) which already contain a complex interplay between two Elements.

By adopting the view just outlined, we are in a position to discuss acupuncture organ-energetic weaknesses or target acupuncture functional units in the same way that behavioral psychology does, making it possible to speak of predisposition to dysfunction with respect to a given reaction pattern.

It may well be, as Requena postulates, that specific types of disorders appear with more frequency in someone whose major reactional mode, for example, brings into play the Water and Fire Elements and the

Greater Yang organ-energetic zones and functions, than in someone whose disturbed energetic zones and functions are different, so that there is (at least from an acupuncture-energetic point of view) a set of basic somatic reaction patterns for each reactive type. Given the complex interplay of the Five Elements (due to the various dynamic cycles that interconnect them all), these basic somatic-energetic reaction patterns might combine in many ways, resulting in an almost infinite variety of reaction patterns that reflect the individuality of each person and situation. Therefore it is untenable to adhere to only Eight Temperaments, thus ignoring the complexity of acupuncture energetics.[32]

If we place the six reaction patterns within the Five Phase diagram, we see the complex series of relationships that arise:

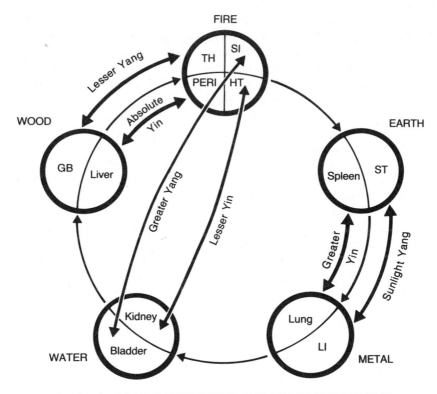

SIX SOMATIC ENERGETIC ZONES AND REACTION PATTERNS

PATTERNS OF AWARENESS AND PATTERNS OF BEHAVIOR

The Five Elements and Twelve Officials as articulated by J. R. Worsley allow us to communicate with an individual from the perspective of his or her own subjective awareness of self, others, and the world. Starting with the Five Element correspondences to the color of the complexion, the sound of the voice, the primary emotional tone, and the pulse, Worsley has developed an approach to acupuncture therapy for the Western practitioner that takes the unique personality of the patient into account. Beginning with an assessment of a person's patterns of awareness, a practitioner will evaluate energetic imbalances in such a way as to contact the person's blocked or unused potential and aid him or her in realizing being-in-the-world in a more complete fashion. In the pages that follow, the reader will find a summary of the Five Elements, viewed on a human scale, and of the Twelve Officials, along with clinical vignettes to illustrate ways in which elemental disturbances may appear in a patient.

The reader will also find personality sketches that result from Requena's view of the Eight Temperaments. The sketches are consistent with character typology and bio-psychology, and combine acupuncture traits with Western morphological bio-types. Following each vignette is a diagram of the somatic energetic reaction zone inherent therein, as I have chosen to reformulate it, with a summary of disorders to which this zone is predisposed.

It must be emphasized that expanding upon the psychological side of acupuncture must be done in a way that remains true to acupuncture-energetic formulations, which display tremendous fluidity and reflect a dynamic perspective and an attitude of relativity.

While the attempt to develop a classification of personality traits and human differences has attracted psychologists throughout history, no such taxonomy has been developed. Most attempts have proved to be of some use, but none has been without flaws. "But the kind of taxonomy on which a science can really build, the kind biologists have known for centuries, is not yet in sight."[33] And why should this surprise us? For human beings are not reducible to some preconceived notion of their biology or behavioral disposition. In working from a bodymind-energetic approach, then, it is important for the practitioner to develop a working hypothesis of a personality theory—deriving as much as possible from his actual clinical experience—that utilizes theories such as Worsley's or Requena's as signposts, not as a master plan.

While Worsley and Requena have developed what appear to be rather complete systems, other practitioners cannot adopt these systems unaltered. Like Worsley and Requena, Western acupuncture therapists, unlike their Oriental counterparts, will always feel the need to understand the personalities of those they treat. We would do well, in this endeavor, to follow the advice of Groddeck, a German physiatrist whose work will be the topic of Chapter 5, who claimed that he constantly developed working hypotheses about the personality configurations and predispositions of his patients and then discarded them when they proved invalid or of no further use.

Following, then, are the working hypotheses of two prominent practitioners of Western acupuncture therapy. In the next chapter, we shall review the classic psychosomatic attempts to solve the bodymind problem, and postulate a bodymind-energetic approach that does not merely expand upon the possible personality theories inherent in traditional acupuncture but juxtaposes acupuncture energetics and Western psychosomatics to forge a decidedly Western approach to the study and practice of energetics.

Five Elements and Twelve Officials—Patterns of Awareness

Beginning from a Taoist perspective that views human beings as an essential part of Nature, the Five Element approach of J. R. Worsley focuses on the role of the Five Elements in human functioning. As Dianne Connelly, an American pioneer of this approach states, "we are the seasons. We are the Elements. Nature is within and without us, each of us every moment. We are a replica of the universe passing from season to season in a natural unending cycle of life."[34]

In practice, this perspective leads to a therapeutic process aimed at achieving harmony in the various elemental functions, both on the somatic level of the energetic-functional units and on the psychological and spiritual levels of the personality, seen as the combination "bodymindspirit." Its major strength lies in its way of developing a deep communication with the person as a complex whole, rather than reducing him or her to a specific imbalance or disease. Focusing on the interplay between the Elements within (the way the energy of Water/Kidneys interrelates with the energy of Fire/Heart, so that the Heart tends to lose control when the Water is low, for example), these practitioners will attempt to discern the Official or Officials (patterns of awareness) that require attention, and direct their acupuncture treatment to a restoration of balance among these Officials. A commonly expressed outcome of this sort of acupuncture therapy is a sense of reintegration of the personality, at times accompanied by a bodily felt sense of well-being. The chief limitation of this approach lies in its unfortunate neglect of the precise meridian-energetic disturbances as they manifest in the body, a definite focus of most other forms of acupuncture therapy. While the energetic restructuring of the personality that occurs in this type of acupuncture therapy may lead to a resolution of specific symptoms or complaints, this approach is not designed for such direct somatic treatment. When practitioners of this approach encounter stubborn somatic-energetic blocks (functional and muscular disorders, for example) they would do well to refer clients to body workers or acupuncture therapists who concentrate more on somatic energetics. In this way, they would afford their clients the possibility of achieving a comprehensive integration of psychological and spiritual changes on the physical level as well.

Utilized as a human-potential therapy focused on self-actualization, the Five Element acupuncture approach introduces the ancient Oriental concept of energetic harmony into the quest for integrity of the personality at all levels, As one looks at the Five Elements and the different personality patterns, or Officials, inherent in each, it becomes immediately apparent how powerful these images of energetic functioning are. While the Five Element therapeutic approach has detailed strategies for effecting energetic transformation on specific levels, an appreciation of these images will also enable other acupuncture therapists, as well as bodyworkers and psychotherapists working in the bodymind-energetic way, to enter into the material, energetic world of the Elements with their clients. This serves to validate the client's inner worlds and results in a client-centered energetic therapy.

PERSONALITY PATTERNS / THE ELEMENTS WITHIN

Fire Element

The Fire Element refers to all that is dynamic, vibrant, excited, and changing. Feeling flushed and overheated, hot with passion, or overflowing with love are all signs of an abundance of Fire. A person with a strong Fire Element will be warm and caring and capable of great enthusiasm and excitement. His or her principle will be the Life principle.[35] A deficiency in the Fire Element, on the other hand, may show up as a lack of enthusiasm or an inability to generate warmth for others. Lacking the energy to embrace life fully, such a person may have great difficulty becoming excited about anything. One may also encounter imbalances in the Fire Element in more complicated contexts—for example, in someone whose Water Element is weak and unable to contain and modulate Fire, resulting in overexcitement, agitation, and a fiery complexion.

The Fire Element is composed of four different personality patterns, known as Officials; the Heart and Heart Protector (both Yin) and the Small Intestine and Triple Warmer (both Yang).[36]

The *Heart Official* is spoken of in the Classics as the monarch who rules through insight and understanding. While this is often interpreted in modern acupuncture as the physiological function of the

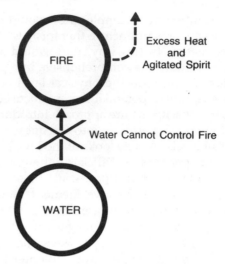

heart pump, Worsley reads this function to mean that the Heart Official, as the "Supreme Controller," oversees the workings of the "bodymindspirit" in order to prevent internal, psychic chaos. Disturbance in this awareness function may lead to erratic thoughts, volatile emotional outbursts, disturbed sleep, and lack of personal warmth, all testifying to a restless spirit.

The *Small Intestine Official* watches over the wealth of the kingdom and is capable of transforming matter (the Alchemist in Worsley's formulation). Known in the Classics as the "Separator of Pure from Impure," (doubtless referring on one level to the role of the small intestine in absorption of nutrients and the passing on of wastes), this can also be understood as the awareness of what is valuable in one's life and the ability to sort out essential emotions, ideas, and values from worthless ones.

The *Pericardium Official*, also known as the "Master of the Heart" or "Heart Protector," occupies the central position of moderating the passions to guard the functioning of the Heart Official, balance the passions and allow for intimacy, and modulate the flow of blood. As such, it is a shock absorber for the Heart, or Supreme Controller, Official.

The *Triple Warmer Official* is the *Official of the Sluices and the Waterways* and is in direct contact with the production of the free-flowing warmth and well-being of the organism. It provides proper thermoregulation on the bodily level and coordination between body, mind, and spirit and within each aspect of the bodymind. When functioning properly, this Official enables one to give and feel the warmth of community and relationship to others.

A CASE OF FIRE LOSS[37]

A shy, humorless man in his 40s came to his acupuncture therapist with a three-year history of cardiac insufficiency. He complained of frightening heart palpitations, newly acquired pains in his sides, and some coughing, occasionally accompanied by bloody sputum. His breathing was rapid and shallow.

Timid and fearful in the interview, the patient blushingly admitted to having been temperamental as a child, frequently crying so hard as to leave himself breathless.[38]

Upon palpation, front and back points associated with the Heart-energetic function were found to be sore. The radial pulses for the Heart function were weak and thin, with some irregularity. The patient's overall facial color was noted as whitish with a lack of red. The therapist was struck by the humorless, serious nature of this man, who reported an incapacity to feel joy. This showed in the sound of his voice, which did not betray the slightest hint of laughter or happiness.

The acupuncture evaluation revealed a deficiency in the Fire Element and the Heart Official, with an inability of the Heart Qi to function normally.

Earth Element

The Earth Element refers not only to the ground on which we stand but also to a sense of being grounded and rooted within ourselves, being at home inside. It is the source of our physical nourishment, and represents our physical connectedness with the planet Earth. All other Elements derive their force from the Earth, in the sense that the Earth is the central Element for human life. Someone with a strong Earth Element will be centered, and well integrated, and will feel at home within himself or herself as well as in the outside world. Such a person is at ease in all situations. A person suffering from a deficiency in this function may tend to become obsessed, looking constantly elsewhere for answers or for support, not realizing that this must come from his or her own center.

A more complex energetic imbalance often associated with a deficiency in Earth arises if the Wood Element is overly active, in which case the Wood functions invade Earth and weaken its ability to be calm and rooted (see diagram on page 88).

The Earth Element is composed of two Officials, the Spleen (Yin) and Stomach (Yang) Officials.

The *Spleen Official* is noted in the classics as the Official in charge of the transportation and transformation functions of the body. This

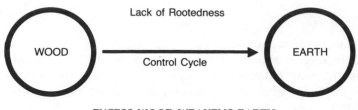

EXCESS WOOD WEAKENS EARTH

is generally taken to mean the absorption, in alliance with the Small Intestine sorting function, of nutrients from food, liquids, and air, and the continual transformation of body fluids. In Worsley's formulation, this is the "Official in Charge of Distribution," the "Energy Transporter," with the role of regulating one's awareness of the center of one's Being—grounding, as it were, the "bodymindspirit" solidly on the Earth. Venturing a comparison with the psychoanalytic perspective, one may associate the Earth Element with the oral stage of psychosexual development, when the world is experienced through the mouth and lips (end points for the circulation of the two Earth pathways of the Stomach and Spleen) and when everything centers on the mother, with issues of nourishment, caring, and love tied to the core of the emerging personality.

The *Stomach Official* is in charge of the public granaries and gives rise to the five tastes (associated with the Five Elements). Worsley refers to this Official as the "Official of Rotting and Ripening," a term that denotes not only the taking in and digesting of food and drink but also the psychological and spiritual ability to assimilate life experiences. It is the Stomach Official who incorporates experiences and processes them, working in intimate relationship with the Spleen Official to ground the personality on a firm basis. Someone with a deficiency in the two Earth Officials will be unable to assimilate experiences and will be devoid of a Center. The two Earth Officials work together— more closely, perhaps, than any other Officials—to stabilize the individual.

A CASE OF EARTHLESSNESS

A pale, somewhat overweight middle-aged woman entered acupuncture treatment complaining of diarrhea, poor appetite, and cold extremities.

Examination revealed a distended abdomen and swollen extremities. The patient's complexion was sallow; her tongue was pale but moist, as were her lips; and her radial pulses were weak and empty, especially in the position associated with Earth.

Her history revealed a great deal of difficulty conceiving, and she reported feeling chronically fatigued since the birth of her only child, a son. She also admitted to very low sexual drive and an almost total absence of feeling most of the time.

Obese as a child, this woman was continually fighting a sweet tooth and attempted to keep her weight down by "starving" herself, "eating bland foods—I guess everything is bland in my life anyway!"[39]

The acupuncture therapist felt that through her monotonous, sing-song litany of vague complaints, this patient was calling for sympathy and warmth, for something to ground her. The above signs and symptoms clearly pointed to a deficiency in the Earth function and the Spleen Official. This weakness made it difficult for her to process and make use of her life experiences and impossible for her to take in and accept the sympathy and emotional warmth she craved.

The Stomach Official was also disturbed, leaving this woman with assimilation problems, affecting her ability to take in food as well as the experiences of her life, and leaving her physically and emotionally starved.

Metal Element

The Metal Element—composed of the Lungs, which take in the Energy from the atmosphere, and the Large Intestine, which aids in the elimination of nonvital and toxic substances—has to do with the ability of the bodymind to take in and let go, energetically and emotionally. The Metal Element is implicated in the orderly circulation of energy (oxygen and blood) throughout the organism, which is why Connelly refers to Metal as a force for conduction and networking, not only in the body but emotionally and psychologically as well.[40]

The first breath of Life depends on the integrity of the Metal Element within us. It is interesting to note the relationship between the diaphragm, which reacts to the severing of the umbilical cord at birth, and the Lungs, which open at that moment to take in the outside world for the first time, for the diaphragm is under the control of the Liver-energetic function and is the last meridian in the circulation of energy. From the region of the diaphragm (where the Liver meridian ends) deep, internal branches spread out into the neck and chest through the esophagus and connect with the energetic functions of the Lungs,where the circulation of energy in the meridians starts up anew. Therefore, the Metal function, via the Lungs, is the function that communicates with the entire circulation of energy through the meridian networks and insures their orderly flow. That which cannot be taken in fully will be expelled by the Metal Element. On the psychological level this might be viewed as the capacity to take in and be with others but also to differentiate oneself from others and stand alone. Metal, in this sense, is the energetic support of the bodymind and gives strength to the Self.

Disorders of Metal will show up on the skin, which is controlled by the Lung-energetic function, in the throat and functions of respiration themselves (coughing, asthma, and bronchitis), and in the functions of elimination (diarrhea and constipation). A person who is weak in the Metal Element will be slow and lethargic, will tend toward depression, will tend to have a lowered resistance—especially in the Fall when he will get a severe cold or flu or bronchitis—and will have a tendency toward general breakdown in communications, physically and emotionally. A more complex disturbance of Metal will occur when Metal is especially weak, resulting in an inability of Metal to control Wood (Liver- and Gallbladder-energetic functions and Officials) along the control cycle of the Five Phases, with a feeling of weakness and pressure in the chest and tightness in the pit of the Stomach (diaphragm), and a concomitant inability to muster the energy necessary to carry out life plans (planning, under the control of the Liver Official, will be impaired owing to lack of energetic control from the Lungs).

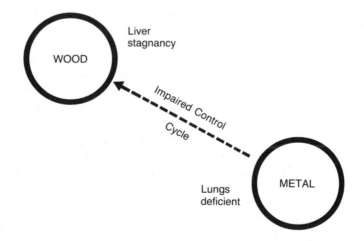

The Metal Element is composed of two Officials, the Lungs (Yin) and the Large Intestine (Yang).

The *Lung Official* is the minister responsible for the orderly circulation of breath and Qi (energy) throughout the organism. Worsley terms this the "Official Who Receives the Pure Energy from the Heavens," which refers not only to the taking in of Air, the "breath of Life" itself, but also to the capacity to breathe in emotional atmospheres completely. Acupuncturists frequently note a loss of vitality and resultant sadness bordering on depression when there is a weakness in this Official's function of fully opening up to take in life. This often is associated with a weakness in the Earth Official's centering and grounding functions, known as a problem of "mother (Earth) and child (Metal)." This is similar to the psychoanalytic conception of the oral stage, which could be likened to the Earth functions of centering the Self and grounding it on a firm basis (what Winnicot terms "adequate mothering"), giving way to a successful transition through the anal stage, similar to the Metal functions of assimilating and eliminating. When these two stages occur properly, the Self will be sufficiently grounded to enable separation from the mother; this leads to appropriate grieving that does not endanger the integrity of the Self, which is able to stand alone. Metal disorders, then, frequently revolve around early childhood experiences in learning to take charge of oneself and one's body (toilet training and muscular control in general). Somatic problems like constipation will arise in connection with difficulty in letting go (of experiences, of others, of a great loss). Respiratory problems, such as asthma, will often be connected to deficiencies in the Metal function of fully taking in, physically by expanding the chest and psychologically by expanding one's heart. Such disorders will show up in people with withdrawn personalities, whose Metal functions do not allow for taking in Life. This will be due either to a deficiency in the capacity to take in (Lung Official) or to a state of being overloaded, emotionally constipated, because of an inability to let go of hurtful past experiences (Large Intestine Official).

The eliminating function of the Large Intestine is under control of the "Official Drainer of the Dregs." By this, Worsley means not only the elimination of wastes, but also the ability to let go emotionally. Emotional constipation (or its opposite, letting "everything hang out") refers back to this Official.

A CASE OF FALL DEPRESSION

One fall a tall, thin, pale young man visited his acupuncturist asking for help with his cough and mild asthma, chronic problems that grew worse each year at that time. He also complained of sweating profusely upon even the mildest exertion, a condition he found disgusting.

The patient reluctantly admitted to bouts of depression in early life but seemed annoyed with the need to discuss "things better forgotten," and proudly stated that he never cried, had no reason to cry, always took care of himself, and needed no one else.

Palpation of the radial pulses revealed a very weak upper heater pulse (associated with the Lung energetic function) as well as pain in the associated front and back points for the Lungs.

At the end of the intake interview, the patient, still clearly annoyed by a procedure that included his psychological history, mentioned that he hadn't cried even at his father's death, which had taken place when the patient was seven years old, and that his mother had always "suffocated" him with her "babying."

The acupuncture evaluation revealed a deficiency in the Metal functions with a primary weakness in the Lung Official and a damming up of the functions of the Large Intestine Official. This weakness, which impaired the man's ability to absorb and eliminate experiences and rendered him emotionally dry (unable to express tears or show grief), showed in deficient Lung Energy. As might be expected, this emotional damming up was often associated with physical constipation as well, leading him to resort to strong purgatives.

Water Element

The Water Element provides the images utilized by the original acupuncturists to describe the flow of energy through the bodymind, with notions such as seas, springs, wells, rivers, and irrigation channels occurring throughout the early texts to denote the flow of energy through the organism. This has led some acupuncture therapists to see acupuncture as the stimulation of electrolytes within the watery substances of the body itself. Since the human body is virtually all water, it is not surprising that the earliest acupuncturists attributed such importance to this Element within.

The Water Element is the Root of Life, with Fire contained within Water—both because Water controls Fire along the control cycle, and because Water is also the spark of Life (with the Bladder conceived as the Battery or energy reserves and the Kidney function known as MingMen or Life Gate Fire). The Water Element is also the source of Will Power. A person with a disturbance on the Water Element will therefore lack the force necessary to accomplish or achieve anything in Life.

A deficiency in the Water Element will lead to a lifelong battle with fatigue, both physical and spiritual, and a person with a severe deficiency in this Element will feel destined never to live fully, and feel haunted by the specter of serious illness. Such persons will often have gradually debilitating diseases.

The Water Element is composed of two Officials, the Kidneys (Yin) and the Bladder (Yang).

The *Kidney Official* is the cornerstone of the constitution, the storehouse of vital energy inherited from one's parents and acquired throughout life. Known as the "Official Who Stores Vital Essence" in Worsley's teachings, this Official is in charge of will power and purposefulness, as mentioned earlier. If this Official is severely disturbed, the defenses of both body and soul will be lowered, leading to disintegration of the spirit and loss of the will to live.

Classically, the *Bladder Official* is thought to store the overflow of fluids and regulate water elimination, as in Western physiology, but in Worsley's conception this "Official in Charge of Eliminating Fluid Wastes" also dictates the bodymind's capacity to adapt to and cope with changing situations. Likened to the battery of a car, this Official provides the emotional reserves necessary to adapt to the flow of life. Connected to the "Small Intestine Official that Separates Pure from Impure" (both constitute the Greater Yang energetic unit), the reserves of the Bladder will make it possible for its connected Official, the Small Intestine, to sort out and prioritize things, thereby rendering smooth adaptation possible.

A CASE OF LACK OF WILL

On a snowy day in January, a quiet, shy man in his 30s with a pallid, greyish complexion came for acupuncture treatment complaining of a constant, dull soreness in his lower back which he said had grown steadily more pronounced over the previous several years. This condition made it impossible for him to do any sort of physical activity, although he had been quite athletic in his youth. Now he grew easily tired. He was found to have cold extremities and was adamant in his dislike of cold weather, which he said "chilled him to the bone." He admitted to waking up several times at night to urinate and experiencing chronic achiness in the pelvic area, which was a constant source of annoyance and concern (even though a medical examination for prostatitis had proved negative).

Lacking ambition, this patient felt no drive and said that each winter he sank into a state of emotional and physical "hibernation." His radial pulses were frail.

The acupuncture evaluation revealed a deficiency in the Water Element, especially the Kidney Official, with a resulting weakness of the Yang (sexual and Fire) Root of the Kidneys, leaving him cold and sexually inactive most of the time.

Wood Element

The Wood Element conjures up the image of Spring and the ability of the bodymind to breathe new life, to be creative and capable of change. Like a tree, a person with a strong Wood Element will be flexible and not lose his or her roots when pressured by Life. Such a person will abound in energy and the will to live (from the mother, the Water Element) and will be able to make complex life decisions, plan ahead, and execute the plans. When an idea takes root in a person with a strong Wood Element, it will germinate and bear fruit.

When disturbed, the Wood Element can give rise to a feeling of being emotionally stuck and to constriction, with muscle twitches and spasms, stiff joints, and a tightness in the diaphragm, chest, and throat.[41]

The Wood Element is composed of two Officials, the Liver (Yin) and Gallbladder (Yang).

The *Liver Official* is the military leader "Who Excels in Strategic Planning." On a physiological-energetic level, this means the ability of the Liver organ to store and make use of nutrients as needed. Worsley emphasizes the more psychological function of the Liver Official in making plans and in creativity, and the classics emphasize the role of the Liver in "promoting the smooth flow of the emotions," keeping one on an even keel.

The *Gallbladder Official*, known as "The Upright Official Who Excels Through Decision and Judgement," regulates the usage of bile at the appropriate time as well as the ability to make appropriate decisions. When this function is seriously disturbed, a person will not be able to make even the smallest decisions.

A CASE OF LIVERISH HEADACHE

A young woman sought acupuncture treatment for frequent, unilateral migraine headaches. The headaches were accompanied by nausea and a bitter taste in her mouth. She also complained of cystic breasts, which became exquisitely tender just before her period, and of severe menstrual pain and dark clotting. In addition, she experienced frequent tightness in her sides and pit of the stomach.

She developed conjunctivitis on two occasions after being out in the wind, and since then had tolerated drafts poorly. Her radial pulses were thin and hard, like a stretched wire, and a bit rapid.

Her emotional life was characterized by constant irritability, with a tendency to hold in her anger for long periods of time and then to unleash it suddenly upon minor provocation. She mentioned in passing that she had great difficulty planning her future, owing to a tendency to be pessimistic and depressed.

The acupuncture evaluation pointed to constraint in the Wood Element's function of maintaining smooth flow through the bodymind, especially the Liver Official. The Gallbladder Official was also found to be disturbed, explaining the migraines' location on the side of the head and temple (the path of the Gallbladder meridian) and the bitter taste in her mouth (and in her life, one might add).

The patient was relieved and intrigued to learn that all of her complaints were part of the same acupuncture-energetic imbalance, namely, a blockage of the Liver-energetic function in the pelvis, stomach, and breasts, as well as the emotional constriction and irritability.

EIGHT ACUPUNCTURE TEMPERAMENTS: BEHAVIOR PATTERNS

Starting with the view that acupuncture is a psychosomatic modality of treatment and influenced by a behavioral, bio-typological framework, Yves Requena has developed a theory of acupuncture personality that expands upon the six energetic units (Greater Yang, Lesser Yin, and so forth), conceptualizing them as Eight Temperaments or personality types, with specific predispositions to disease in each.

While such a concept may tend to freeze the dynamic acupuncture-energetic framework into the still shots of character typing, it does provide a new perspective from which to view acupuncture therapy in the West, and serves as a point of departure for discussing acupuncture personality predispositions to disease.

Focusing on the dynamics of the great meridians (Greater Yang, Lesser Yin, and so on), some French acupuncturists have arrived at a very sophisticated approach to acupuncture therapeutics that begins with what might be termed somatic energetic repatterning.

Requena's use of the six great meridians, expanded into Eight Temperaments to correspond with the eight bio-typological temperaments (Corman, Berger) begins with an assessment of a person's body type (and temperamental correlations to it).

Once this is determined, it is possible to understand many if not all of the patient's complaints and disorders as manifestations of a disturbance in the somatic-energetic reaction patterns characteristic of this type. This enables the therapist to grasp the unity of the disparate disturbances and initiate treatment to restore more appropriate responses in this zone.

Starting with the body, Requena develops a form of treatment that is capable of reintegrating body and mind.

Whereas Worsley's approach ignores the complexity of the somatic acupuncture-energetic dynamics, Requena's approach retrieves a fundamental understanding of the meridian energetics. This leads to a meridian-energetic acupuncture, similar in many respects to various Japanese and Korean formulations, that affirms the primacy of the meridian network. Such approaches are powerful short-term therapies for many structural and functional disorders, as well as psychosomatic complaints.

In the pages that follow, we shall provide the reader with quick vignettes of each of the Eight Temperaments, to illustrate the character typing inherent in Requena's approach. Each vignette will be followed by a graphic representation of this temperament as a somatic energetic zone with the major symptoms of the somatic energetic reaction patterns pertaining to it. For a detailed discussion of the predisposition to disease in each zone/temperament, see Requena's works listed in the bibliography.

Greater Yang Temperament (Small Intestine-Bladder/Fire-Water)

High-strung, rebellious, and acutely sensitive to criticism, the Greater Yang child learns in adulthood to hide his or her tense nature and violent emotions and adopts a distant, condescending attitude toward others. With a noble, proud appearance, piercing glance, and faultless memory for past events and slights, such a person is likely to be labeled a snob, often feels rejected, unfairly judged, or misunderstood.

The Greater Yang person may embrace causes with a passion so great as to verge on fanaticism, and may find it difficult to admit to possible error. This person's relationships can be stormy and dramatic, as he or she is a possessive, jealous, and authoritarian lover.

The Greater Yang type is articulate, persuasive, and honorable to duty.

Such an individual may be a fitful sleeper. Vulnerable to convulsions, epilepsy, and nosebleeds as a child, this person as an adult will suffer from illnesses that always are acute or explosive, and will follow a treatment plan only if a close relationship with the doctor exists.

Lesser Yang Temperament (Gallbladder-Triple Heater/Wood-Fire)

Strong, muscular and agile, the olive-skinned Lesser Yang individual takes in the world through large, deep-set, piercing eyes. He or she is rarely sick in childhood and adolescence, barring an occasional migraine or bout with liver trouble. Though athletic, such a person may have difficulty rotating sideways (stiffness of the Belt Channel, fed by the Gallbladder meridian); tend to retire late in the evening, sleep late, and rise slowly; hate the wind and drafts; be indifferent to cold; and have strong feelings one way or the other about heat. The Lesser Yang individual has a good memory that may deteriorate in mid-life.

Untiring, optimistic, and full of plans and future projects, this type of person always is on the move, likes to work, craves challenges, is committed totally to the work at hand, and always feels that time is too short. The person feels capable but often will not know how to approach a task; this may lead to a lack of coherence at times.

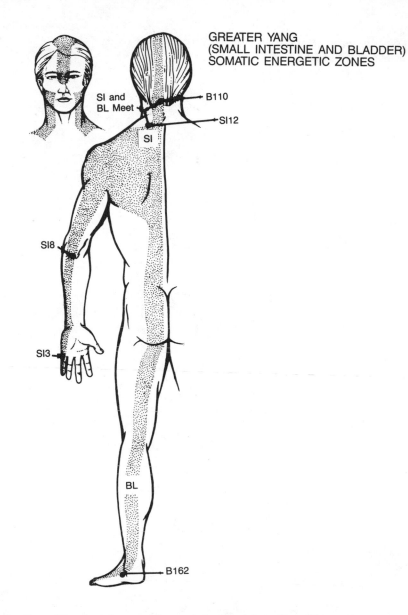

GREATER YANG
(SMALL INTESTINE AND BLADDER)
SOMATIC ENERGETIC ZONES

SI and BL Meet

B110

SI12

SI

SI8

SI3

BL

B162

Dysfunctions: stiff neck, tightness of the cervical region (where SL and BL meridians meet) and spine (SI3 governs the governing vessel); high blood pressure, constipation, diarrhea, Crohn's disease; urinary and prostate complaints; impotence, amenorrhea; Cushing's syndrome; ankylosing spondylarthritis; epilepsy, convulsions, vertigo, vertical occipital headaches, insomnia; psoriasis, eczema, acne on the forehead and upper back (SI and BL zones); paranoia, paranoid depressive states. Bladder Meridian "sciatica."*

Key Points: SI3, BL62, SI12, BL10.

*CF. Requena, Terrains and Pathology in Chinese Medicine. Brookline, Massachusetts: Redwing, 1985.

97

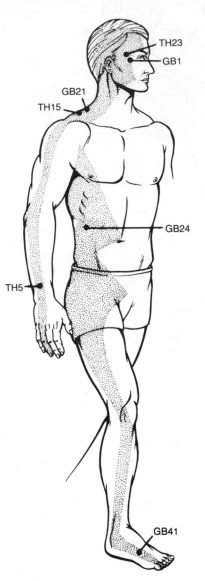

Dysfunctions: high blood pressure, stiff Belt Channel and lower back, difficulty rotating, varicose veins, phlebitis, stomach ulcers, constipation, hemorrhoids, arthritis (gouty), gall and kidney stones, facial muscle twitches or neuralgias, sweating disorders, clenched jaws, mandibular arthritis, arthritis of the hip joint, lateral sciatica.

Key Points: TH5, GB41, GB21, TH15, GB1, TH23.

Generous, cordial, friendly, and enthusiastic, the Lesser Yang individual occasionally may get into trouble by being too frank and open. He or she may become belligerent or violent when angry, but the anger dissipates quickly. Such a person is incapable of holding a grudge and cannot bear family quarrels or legal battles.

In love matters, this person can be open to several lovers, without holding back on any.

Anxiety, this person's greatest weakness, can be touched off by minor events. The Lesser Yang individual does not like to be sick and does not like to be taken care of. Overall, this person's strength is in activity: in the ability to make decisions and act on them.

Earth Sunlight Yang Temperament (Stomach)

The individual of Earth Sunlight Yang Temperament is balanced and centered: always broadly built and wide at the shoulders and hips, with a short neck and fleshy, sometimes obese, body. The person never plays sports for health but only for pleasure.

The expression is soft and innocent, though the eyes can show many emotions ranging from joy to malice.

Childhood health is good, though the person may have some nose and throat problems in winter that will disappear in adolescence. The person eats a lot, has a sweet tooth, may become obese in pre-puberty, and later may suffer from sinusitis and acquire a red and congested complexion.

The Earth Sunlight Yang person has a good memory but tends to make use of mnemonic devices. He or she likes intellectual games, word puzzles, puns, and riddles, and remembers tactics and strategies for winning, both at games and at politics.

This person shows initiative and is practical, observant, liberal, polite, ironic, skeptical, and spirited. Basically non-emotional and extroverted, he or she downplays everything and thus appears objective. Other people often see this individual as comforting, reassuring and amusing, which is a mistake because the person is not especially aware of others' needs.

The person with an Earth Sunlight Yang Temperament is very sensual but superficial in love affairs, does not have a tragic outlook on life, and may lack tact.

He or she has a happy disposition but may suffer from too much optimism (like spending money without having it). Though social success is important, such a person is not very ambitious or willing to make big sacrifices, but will grasp opportunity if it happens to knock.

Illnesses come late in life and almost always are due to excesses. This person is hard to treat because of the high priority on enjoyment.

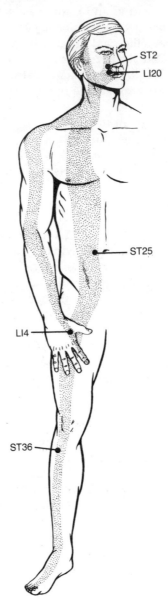

Dysfunctions: high blood pressure, cardiac disorders, mania, asthma, hiatus hernia, nausea, dyspepsia, vomiting, loss of appetite, colitis, constipation, hypothyroidism, shin splints, weakness, excessive hunger, eating disorders.

Key Points: ST36, LI4, ST25, LI20, ST2.

Metal Sunlight Yang Temperament (Large Intestine)

The person possessing a Metal Sunlight Yang Temperament is balanced, has long, refined features, and may have beauty marks all over the body. With age, this person may become heavy or thin, with dry skin and plentiful wrinkles. The facial expression is clear, confident, and calm, though anxiety may cause grimacing.

This person may be either thin or heavy in childhood, but if heavy will often become suddenly thin at adolescence. Bronchitis, nose and throat problems, asthma, and constipation may occur in childhood.

This type of person enjoys a good memory, prefers abstract systems of thought like mathematics, and is active but rigid, non-emotional, cool, and indifferent. It is virtually impossible to upset the person, who therefore often appears distinguished.

He or she respects rules and principles, keeps promises, has a deep sense of civic duty to any collectivity, and has a strong respect for the law.

The person of this temperament has good health as an adult but may develop colitis, and when ill, gives his or her body to the doctor like a car to the garage mechanic.

Earth Greater Yin Temperament (Spleen)

The Earth Greater Yin type is round—round in face and shoulders, and round in gestures, with a pale, milky or peachy complexion; soft skin; and little body hair. This type of person is not very agile, has a gentle, calm, peaceful, and joyous expression, can adapt to all climates except humidity, and does not overexert himself or herself for anything, ever.

In childhood such a person will be goodnatured and overweight, having an excessive appetite and a sweet tooth. Problems include earaches, bronchitis, bedwetting, and slow descent of the testicles or late onset of menstruation.

As an adult this type will get temporarily tired at 11 A.M. and 5 P.M. and will use sweets for energy.

Though able to pick up the nuances of an argument, the Earth Greater Yin type tends to be somewhat absent-minded and distractable, and when tired to have the sensation that the head is not working and that thought and concentration are impossible.

Non-emotional and non-active, this person might be called a passive extrovert, fond of socializing but unlikely to seek contacts actively. Good-natured and mild-mannered, he or she is a good listener, will not impose ideas on others, is tolerant to the point of being indifferent, and is not upset by aggressiveness in others. When faced with conflict, this person will not oppose, but will just wait, exhibiting a passive stubbornness. He or she remains untouched by most events and has no interest in the past. This type has no ambition and is lazy and negligent, but is often seen by others as a practical philosopher, and can make use of this attribute successfully.

This type is never in a rush, is always late but never feels guilty about it, and can get carried away by impulses, especially in art, music, and the theater.

The Earth Greater Yin Temperament can replace a deep, loving relationship with a mediocre one and claim that it is just as profound.

This person can become very depressed. When this occurs, mental functions are lost, ideas don't flow logically, and the person feels incapable of doing the slightest thing. He or she will then become isolated, and the only activity will be eating. Obesity may be a problem.

Metal Greater Yin Temperament (Lungs)

This person is narrow in the shoulders and chest; has long, thin features and slow movements; and may be either blond, blue-eyed and pale[43] with a steely, often frightening distant stare, or a brown-haired, dark-eyed person with a hard glance who never forgives and inspires no confidence or trust.

This type may have difficult or shallow breathing and can garner energy only by resting. He or she dislikes humidity and cold.

Weak, fragile, pale, easily tired, and having a poor appetite in childhood, this type suffers from respiratory disturbances or constipation, and skin disorders like eczema and psoriasis.

In adulthood, the person is always tired and worn out, feels that energy will never be regained, needs lots of rest and vacations, goes to sleep early, and rises early.

The Metal Greater Yin type conserves energy in gestures, moves slowly, and talks slowly with an effort, as if forcing the voice farther than it wants to go. This person is meticulous, has a good sense of judgment, and is on time, but is also apathetic and introverted, and tends to ruminate over the past. He or she is often judgmental and can be bitter, reacts to conflicts with inertia, can be stubborn, and is solitary and closed off. If not totally absorbed, this person will go off on flights of imagination and will feel that time is frozen. Feeling that time moves very slowly, he or she will become easily bored and anxious.

Such a person is hostile to change, organizes life in advance, doesn't like to improvise, is a slave of habit, and likes order and discipline.

Though always honest, this person will never go straight for something. He can be thrifty or cheap.

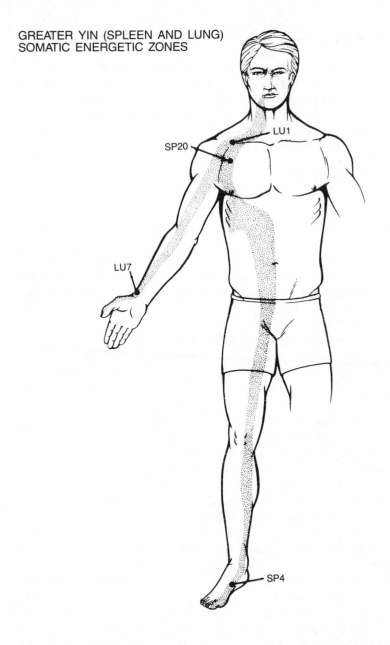

Dysfunctions: Disorders of respiratory tract, sore throat, frequent colds, asthma, pleurisy, emphysema, bradycardia, Raynaud's syndrome, disorders of vessels, gastric disorders, intestinal complaints, pancreatitis, nephrotic syndromes, cystitis, prostatitis, all menstrual disorders, hypothyroidism, diabetes, obesity, degenerative arthritis and rheumatoid arthritis, headaches, convulsions, acne, eczema, psoriasis, collagen diseases, Hodgkin's disease, sinusitus, farsightedness, obsessional neurosis, depressive states, schizophrenia.

Key Points: SP4, LU7, LU1, SP20.

He or she is a precise talker with a tendency to split hairs, but does go off on tangents or sprinkle comments with drawn-out footnotes.

This type is compassionate, understanding, and forgiving.

Such a person is often treated medically for one thing or another and will follow treatment plans.

The two Greater Yin types often overlap.

Absolute Yin Temperament (Liver-Pericardium/Wood-Fire)

Attractive, with large, expressive eyes and a cloudy, far-off expression, the Absolute Yin individual is often seen by others as mysterious and alluring.

Though usually nervous, moody, timid, and inhibited, this type can be talkative, emotional, and excited among friends and when defenses are down. When inhibited, the person may bite the nails, have behavioral tics, and blush easily. It is the eyes that betray anxiety, fatigue, and inhibition.

Such a person is healthy in childhood except for liver crises, or indigestion and nausea or vomiting. He or she faints easily, dislikes needles and the sight of blood or any strong odor, and often has a fear of heights. Requena states that those suffering from myopia (nearsightedness) are always Absolute Yin.

This type dislikes the wind, often experiencing vertigo, confusion, or bad temper when exposed to it, and likes spring best, although it often brings with it a feeling of malaise.

He or she has a poor memory for things of little personal interest; and consequently may have large gaps in the memory.

The Absolute Yin type is unstable and moody: emotional, nervous, non-active, and a bit hysterical. Anxiety can be brought on by almost anything, and is reacted to by shutting down. In women the menstrual cycle may be accompanied by depression and anxiety (premenstrual syndrome).

A person of this temperament works only intermittently and can do only enjoyable things. He or she creates a mask to face the outside world, and takes refuge internally, which others may find seductive.

Though timid and anxious, this person can be exhibitionistic and is subject to emotional rages. He or she likes to have fun and to get lost in activities like reading books.

This type is often addicted to coffee, tea, or tobacco, and can easily get nauseated and develop migraines. The person may be sick frequently, usually not seriously, and usually will not follow treatment or cooperate with a treatment plan.

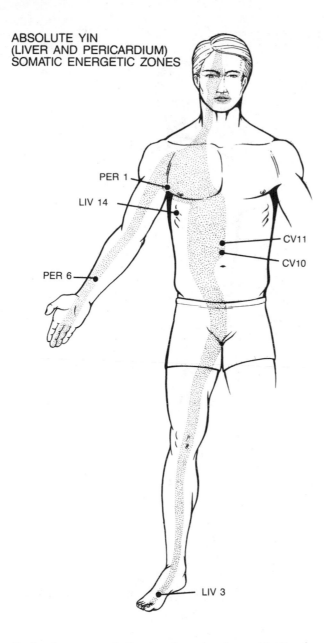

ABSOLUTE YIN
(LIVER AND PERICARDIUM)
SOMATIC ENERGETIC ZONES

PER 1

LIV 14

CV11

CV10

PER 6

LIV 3

Dysfunctions: seasonal allergic asthma, hay fever, skin disorders, tachycardia, palpitations, labile hypertension, varicose veins, phlebitis, circulatory paresthesias, chronic liver disorders, bilious vomiting, right-sided colitis, viral hepatitis, cystitis (transitory) dysmenorrhea with cystic breasts, fibroids, premenstrual syndrome, hot flashes, hyperthyroidism, frontal and orbital headaches, migraines, vertigo, dystonia, cramps and spasms, hives, acne, acute dermatitis, conjuctivitis, myopia, anxiety, hysteria, outbursts of anger.

Key Points: LIV3, PER6, LIV14, CV10, CV11, PER1.

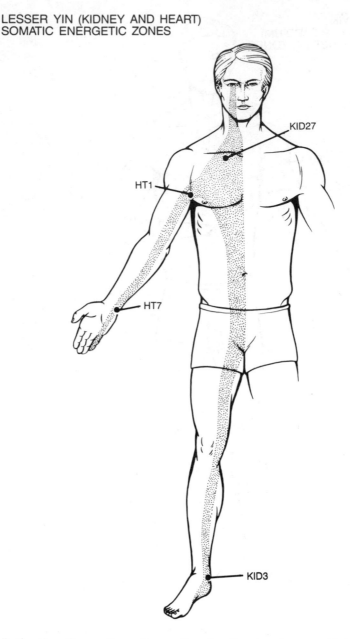

Dysfunctions: Raynaud's syndrome, all cardiac disorders, hypo- and hypertension, arteriosclerosis, constipation, bladder infections, renal diseases, edema, prostate disorders, chronic genitourinary disorders, adrenal insufficiency, juvenile diabetes, degenerative arthritis, ankylosing spondylarthritis, meningitis, Parkinsons's disease, warts, acne, lupus erythematosus (with Greater Yin), hearing and ear disorders, keratitis, depressive states, melancholia.

Key Points: HT7, KID3, HT1, KID27.

Lesser Yin Temperament (Heart-Kidney/Fire-Water)

The introverted Lesser Yin type moves rapidly with a timid clumsiness. The back is curved, the head lowered, and the person looks down while walking. The expression is sad, as though the person has just been crying. He or she is easily chilled, hates the heat or cold, hibernates in the winter, and often has reddish cheeks and blushes easily, though the complexion turns gray during illness.

This individual has fragile health and is prone to sore throats and earaches. Childhood arthritis may occur, chronic lumbar disorders are common, and old age almost always brings rheumatism. This type can easily be paired with another temperament.

The person is dependent on the past and remembers it easily, but otherwise the memory is faulty. He or she cannot learn by rote and has a conceptual, not practical, intelligence.

Emotional, sentimental, and meditative, this person doesn't like to make great efforts. Though conscientious, he or she always feels defeated in advance, and is full of humility, discreet, and honest. This type tends toward melancholy, feeling that life is absurd and effort useless, and often questions the meaning of life but is not suicidal.

The Lesser Yin type leans heavily toward self-analysis, keeps secret diaries, is well aware of personal weaknesses, will yearn for self-improvement, and is often masochistic. He or she values intimacy and in relationships will have an all-or-nothing attitude, is very faithful in love relationships, has absolute ideals of what one should be like, and wants perfection. This person is jealous and totally destroyed by infidelity, and cannot love easily a second time.

Such a person is energized by intimacy with nature, a loved one, or friendship.

Because of constitutional weaknesses, the Lesser Yin type is prey to serious and chronic illnesses, but is aware of this, and so lives life cautiously.

CHAPTER SUMMARY

The Chinese medical model takes the psychological life of the individual into account only to the extent that correspondences exist between each of the Five Elements and a temperamental and emotional disposition. This is not surprising, since the Chinese notion of the individual is social rather than psychological, and a "psychological subject" does not have to be accounted for. The result is that a patient in China will tend to somatize emotional experiences with no outlet for expressing their significance. In contrast, Western patients often enter acupuncture therapy having already made associations between their physical problems and their psychological states. Therefore, the Western practitioner must take the psychological being of the patient into account if more than symptomatic acupuncture is to be attempted.

The Chinese medical classics offer little for those who want to expand the scope of acupuncture to include understanding and communication with the patient on the psychological level. This may be why two European practitioners, J. R. Worsley and Yves Requena, felt compelled, while beginning with traditional sources, to develop approaches to acupuncture therapy that included an acupuncture psychology or acupuncture personality theory.

Worsley's concept of the Five Element constitutions and Twelve Officials retrieves an anthropomorphized, humanized view of the twelve organ-energetic functions, attributing to each a particular personality configuration (Official) that presides over it. The functions of the Officials, mentioned fleetingly in the Chinese medical classics, are expanded upon by Worsley to create a psychological profile. These functions represent inherited or early learned potentials and limitations, with the constitutional factors being the aspect of the bodymind that has both the predisposition to dysfunction and also the greatest potential. Intervention here, on the side of the psyche, involves working at a deep level for a long time. In this sense, Worsley's approach is psychoenergetic and more appropriate for issues of quality of life and self-actualization than for treatment of specific physical complaints or disorders.

Requena's Eight Temperaments are inherited or early learned somatic-energetic reaction patterns, called into play by a weakness or imbalance in one of six energetic zones of the bodymind. These personality configurations develop through reaction to the environment somatically, with all of the peculiarities, potentials, and limitations of the body itself (somatic compliance).

My hypothesis here is that a somatic-energetic reaction pattern shields the deeper core constitutional elemental imbalance.[44] This view invites intervention more on the "side of the soma."

Requena has analyzed Western categories of disease, taking account of their association with the Five constitutions and the Eight temperaments, by grouping them into the six greater meridian-energetic systems. In this way, body type, easily ascertained by an assessment of which energetic zones are involved in a given individual and situation, can be evaluated, and treatment of disorders can begin with a recognition of somatic constitutional predispositions.

This approach provides a way of viewing target organs and predisposition to disease in a new light, and constitutes a somatic-energetic approach capable of intervening in a multiplicity of functional, psychosomatic, and organic disorders in a precise way that takes the uniqueness of the individual at that time into account.

NOTES

1. Capra, *The Turning Point*, pp. 318–319.
2. Cf. *Culture and Self*, especially the Introduction, pp. 2–23.
3. In the past, they would have been referred to an elder.
4. Ibid, p. 14.
5. Cf. *Encounters with Qi*, by Dr. Eisenberg, New York, 1987, for clear examples, in his case histories, of the absence of the psychological subject in Chinese clinics.
6. Cf. *Culture and Self*, especially the Introduction and p. 23.
7. Not that symptomatic relief is a bad thing, to the contrary. A worker with a sprained hand, or an athlete or dancer with a painful back, wants fast, effective relief, and acupuncture is often of significant value here, without the negative side effects of often unnecessary surgery or drugs. A bodymind-energetic perspective would start with the immediate painful or dysfunctional symptoms but would move on to redress deeper imbalances that cut across psychological, physical, and spiritual levels, even in such cases as these.
8. This movement has been exemplified by practitioners trained by Professor J. R. Worsley in Leamington Spa, England, and especially in America in the Traditional Acupuncture Institute, headed by Robert Duggan and Dianne Connelly, who trained with Worsley over a decade ago and have reoriented the training in their institute to form what might be termed a human potential school of traditional acupuncture. A similar experience, starting from the side of the soma and moving toward the side of the psyche, has been implicit in my formulation of training at the Tri-State Institute of Traditional Chinese Acupuncture in Stamford, Connecticut, which I direct. This type of experience is eloquently described by Eric Stephens, speaking of his own development, in *The Journal of Traditional Acupuncture*, Volume VIII, Autumn 1985, pp. 16–19.
9. Ibid, p. 17.
10. Ibid, p. 19.
11. Cf. S. Stansfeld Sargent and Kenneth R. Stafford, *Basic Teachings of the Great Psychologists*. Garden City, New York, Doubleday, 1965, pp. 211–212.
12. Cf. Henry Gleitman, *Psychology*. New York, W. W. Norton, 1981, pp. 645–654; and Leona E. Tyler, *The Psychology of Human Differences*. New York, Appleton-Century-Crofts, 1965, pp. 437–446.
13. Wilheim Reich, *Character Analysis*, 3rd edition. New York, Touchstone Books, Simon & Schuster, 1972, p. 338.
14. Ibid, p. 341.
15. For a fascinating discussion of this more and more problematic encounter, see Edward Shorter, *Bedside Manners: The Troubled History of Doctors and Patients*. New York, Simon Schuster, 1985.
16. J. R. Worsley, a physical therapist and acupuncturist, is the founder of the College of Traditional Chinese Acupuncture in Leamington Spa, England, and founder of the English tradition of Five Element Acupuncture; Yves Requena is a physician who works in Aix-en-Provence, France, a student of Dr. Nguyen Van Nghi and founding president of the Group for Study and Research in Acupuncture.

17. This "humanized" phenomenological view of the Five Elements is presented by Dianne M. Connelly, Ph.D., M.Ac., Dipl.Ac., a student of Worsley, in *Traditional Acupuncture: The Law of the Five Elements,* Centre for Traditional Acupuncture, Columbia, Maryland, and stems from traditional, Taoist concepts of the Five Elements; this approach is strikingly similar to that of the phenomenologists, who stress that a "phenomenological analysis has to consider the distribution and relative predominance of the four elements—fire, air, water, earth—in the patient's subjective worlds," in *Existence,* p. 115.

18. Cf. *Existence,* 115–117, for a discussion and further references to Bachelard's books on a phenomenology of fire, earth, water, and air.

19. Binswanger, "The Existential Analysis School of Thought" in *Existence,* p. 192.

20. As summarized by Ellenberger, "Psychiatric Phenomenology and Existential Analysis," in *Existence,* p. 116.

21. Cf. Ted J. Kaptchuk, *The Web That Has No Weaver: Understanding Chinese Medicine,* pp. 351–352 and "Acupuncture in the West" in *The Journal of Chinese Medicine,* p. 25.

22. Co-founders of the Traditional Acupuncture Institute in Columbia, Maryland, on the basis of Worsley's teachings but with a unique human potential orientation quite their own.

23. Cf. "Homing," an excerpt from Dianne Connelly, *All Sickness Is Homesickness* in *The Journal of Traditional Acupuncture,* Volume VIII, No. 2, Autumn 1985, pp. 26–29.

24. Cf. Anthony Stevens, *Archetypes: A Natural History of the Self.* New York, William Morrow & Co., 1983, p. 27.

25. In *Existence,* p. 192.

26. Cf. Robert Duggan, M.A., M.Ac., "Beyond Symptoms." *Journal of Traditional Acupuncture,* Volume VIII, No. 2, p. 8–9.

27. The procedure Requena uses to draw broad similarities among the concepts of Menetrier, Berger and very brief Chinese descriptions of certain personality traits in the *Ling Shu* is beyond the scope of this book. The reader is referred to Yves Requena, *Terrains and Pathology in Acupuncture.* Brookline, Massachusetts, Paradigm Publications, Redwing Books, 1986, Part 3, Chapter 1 on "The Five Constitutions & Six Temperaments"; and Requena, *Acupuncture et Psychologie: Pour une Approche Nouvelle de la Psycho-Somatique.* Paris, Maloine, 1982, pp. 86–93, 159–238.

28. Requena develops his rationale, quickly and with sometimes hasty correlations, in *Acupuncture et Psychologie,* pp. 87–96 and 159–183.

29. The "emotive" is quick to become excited; the "non-emotive," slow; the "active" readily acts on impulses; the "non-active" delays action; the "primary" reacts in and to the present; the "secondary" reacts in and to the past, as if predetermined by it. The reader will note that "active" is equivalent to *Yang* and "non-active" to *Yin,* and that the emotive types are those within the Fire Element in Requena's formulation.

30. The reader will note that in order to make the eight temperaments of Berger correlate with the six "energetic types" of acupuncture, Requena divided the Earth-Metal Types (Sunlight Yang and Greater Yin), into the EARTH and the METAL types within these larger categories. This is another example of a kind of *forcing* to make correlations fit. Another example is when Requena "reconstitutes" Absolute Yin and Sunlight Yang "types," not given in the Chinese Classics.

31. Cf. *Terrains and Pathology,* Part 3, Chapters 3–5.

32. Why would there not also be a Fire-Earth type, or a Metal-Wood type, etc., in Requena's formulation of it?

33. Gleitman, *Psychology,* p. 653.

34. Dianne Connelly, *Traditional Acupuncture: The Law of The Five Elements.* Columbia, Maryland, Traditional Acupuncture Centre, 1979, p. 13; all references to the Five Elements and Twelve Officials come from this text.

35. Ibid, p. 43.
36. Developed by Worsley from Chapter 8 of the *Yellow Emperor's Classic of Internal Medicine*, Ilza Veith, translator. Berkeley, University of California Press, 1972.
37. Each of the cases in this section is a compilation from several actual cases to better portray each Element and serve as a working image of the Elements in distress.
38. Requena points out this tendency in childhood of the Fire "constitution" to exaggerated emotional outbursts with crying spells and an acute sensitivity to reproach. Cf. *Acupuncture et Psychologie.*
39. Again, Requena notes this childhood tendency in the Earth "Constitution" to obesity and a sweet tooth.
40. Cf. Connelly, *Traditional Acupuncture,* pp. 81–82.
41. Requena notes the frequency of food allergies, especially to eggs and chocolate; nearsightedness; neo-natal jaundice; and viral hepatitis as disorders of a child suffering from a Wood Element imbalance.
42. Cf. Requena, *Terrains and Pathology in Acupuncture.* Brookline, Massachusetts, Paradigm Publications, 1986.
43. The racial overtones of such rigid bio-typing as Requena's is clearly evident in such descriptions as this.
44. For a fascinating alternative, but in certain ways very similar, reading of the six Somatic Energetic Reaction Zones, cf. Stanley Keleman, *Emotional Anatomy,* in which he develops the concept of a dynamic interplay between an external and an internal manner of somatic being-in-the-world.

4

Classic Psychosomatics and the New Bodymind Energetics

> The problem of psychogenesis is linked with the ancient dichotomy of psyche versus soma. Psychological and somatic phenomena take place in the same organism and are merely two aspects of the same process.[1]
>
> F. Alexander

While the attempts to develop acupuncture personality theories discussed in Chapter 3 are exemplary in establishing bases for a properly Western acupuncture therapy, we need not ignore the Western psychological literature, rich in psychosomatic observations, dating from Freud and Groddeck to current investigations of stress as it affects psyche and soma.

In juxtaposing acupuncture energetics, which combines thousands of years of somatic-energetic observations and methodologies, with classic and modern psychosomatics, Western acupuncture therapists and psychotherapists alike will benefit from each other's understanding of bodymind interaction. The introduction of energetics into the discussion of psychosomatic phenomena leads to a *bodymind energetic* method of approach.

With the emergence of a new paradigm of health and healing embodying a truly holistic perspective, the need for an appropriate theory of energy is keenly felt. The Western medical model may well be the only one in history that has not put forth an energetic concept of health and disease. All other healing systems are based on a philosophy of energy or vital force.[2]

The Chinese medical model is by far the most elaborately articulated therapeutic system developed on the basis of energetic balance. Here individual forces are seen as a microcosm of cosmic ones, with correspondences between the forces working in an individual—mind and body—and the forces at work in the Universe. Therefore, a doctor's task in Chinese medicine is to help the individual reestablish a more appropriate balance with external forces. In Chinese medicine, as Capra states, "the ideal doctor is a sage who treats each patient on an individual basis; whose diagnosis does not categorize the patient as having a specific disease but records as fully as possible the individual's total state of mind and body and its relation to the natural and social environment."[3]

But in developing a truly holistic approach to health in the West, it is important to know which aspects of the Chinese model are adaptable to our own context and whether, indeed, the Chinese model is holistic.

Capra points out that the term "holistic" has two meanings. In the first sense, a holistic view depicts the human organism "as a living system whose components are all interconnected and interdependent."[4] Chinese medicine is definitely holistic in this sense. But in a larger sense, "holistic" implies recognition that the living human system is an integral part of larger physical and social systems, "that is constantly affected by the environment but can also act upon it and modify it."[5] In this sense the Chinese model is holistic only in theory. While the classical texts do seem to place equal weight on factors from the external environment, internal emotional states, diet, and the nature of one's life, practitioners of Oriental medicine in the East, and many in the West, "make no practical attempt to deal with the psychological and social aspects of illness therapeutically."[6]

Indeed, a practitioner of Oriental medicine or acupuncture often asks probing questions about the nature of the patient's work, reaction to different types of weather, emotional reactions, life style, sexual drive, and so on, but in treatment chooses acupuncture points or other modalities of treatment to narrowly "manipulate processes inside the body."[7] The Chinese model of the body includes the psychic dimension (tendency to anger, difficulty making decisions, and the like) as part of the body process, yet the fact remains that few practitioners of classical Oriental medicine today seriously take the psychology of the individual into account when arriving at an energetic diagnosis.

While the medical classics of China did espouse a holistic viewpoint of man, nature, medicine, and their interaction, actual practice now (and probably in the past) is narrowly focused on bodily changes. Like the Western medical model it has so openly adopted, Chinese traditional medical practice is fundamentally somatic, privileging the health of the body above that of the mind. In this sense, then, the Oriental medical model also suffers from a mind/body split that neglects, on any practical level, the role of the psyche.

There is a more serious flaw in the Oriental medical model as it concerns our attempts in the West to develop a new paradigm of health and health maintenance. This is, as we saw in Chapter 3, that the primacy of the individual as we know it in the West is replaced by that of the social group. As Capra states, ". . . the Chinese system was probably never very holistic as far as the psychological and social aspects of illness are concerned. The reluctance to act therapeutically by affecting the patient's social situation was certainly a result of the strong influence of Confucianism on all aspects of Chinese life."[8]

Ted Kaptchuk, when teaching Oriental medical concepts to his Western students, found that he had to do more than merely translate the Chinese views wholesale; he also had to present an entirely new cultural view of health and illness. In doing so, he came to realize that on the one hand, while the Oriental model may appear extraordinary to a Westerner, it is "just the ordinary not understood or experienced,"[9] and on the other, that the Western viewpoint has its own share of extraordinariness.

An honest attempt to develop new conceptual models of healing appropriate to our age and culture must also entail an affirmation of areas where the Western approach is more advanced.

DYNAMIC MEDICINE

While the term "psychosomatic" is currently used by the general population as well as many health and mental health professionals to denote the unreal nature of a complaint, a major principle of the new paradigm of health is that *all illness is psychosomatic*. Once we realize that psychosomatic merely means "mind/body," we see that "to say all illness is psychosomatic is to say only that all illness has both physical and mental components."[10]

The term "psychogenic" is the proper term for a psychologically induced physical complaint, whereas "psychosomatic" merely implies bodymind interrelatedness.

The father of American psychosomatics, Franz Alexander, defined psychosomatics as an approach to research and therapy that involves "the simultaneous and co-ordinated use of somatic . . . methods and concepts on the one hand, and psychological methods and concepts on the other."[11] In speaking of the psychosomatic approach in use at the Chicago Institute for Psychoanalysis, which he headed in the 1950s, Alexander referred to it as a "functional," "dynamic," "holistic" medicine that integrates observations of the role of the psyche with those relating to the body and its complex processes. The bodymind energetic approach, then, seeks a revival of this *dynamic, functional* perspective, where the term "energetic" is introduced in order to underscore a view of the bodymind consistent with both the new advances of physics and the age-old acupuncture-energetic perspective, of the body as a force field directly connected to society and the forces of nature.

In exploring three Western psychological attempts to grapple with the body/mind dilemma—from the classic psychosomatic approach inspired by psychoanalytic concepts, through the experiential approach that came to be known as phenomenological psychology, to modern behavioral theories of stress—we wish to provide Western therapists of mind and body alike with a renewed respect for the Western efforts at understanding the complex role of the psyche and psychoenergetics in generating somatic-energetic, functional, and organic disorders.

In his excellent critical survey of psychoanalytically inspired psychosomatics, Günter Ammon emphasizes that there are many approaches to the concept of psychosomatics within psychoanalytic circles,[12] which we shall explore only insofar as they bear on the relationship between psyche and soma in the generation of bodily complaints. The reader interested in the pertinence of the psychosomatic question to psychoanalytic theory and the practice of psychoanalysis is referred to Ammon's study.

THE PSYCHOSOMATIC PROBLEM

The fundamental problem for the pioneers of psychosomatic medicine was the disparity between the *theory* of psychoanalysis, which they selected as their starting point for understanding the genesis of psychosomatic symptoms, and the *practice* of psychoanalysis, which seemed inadequate in resolving the actual physiological mechanism at work in such disorders. While psychoanalytic theory was of great value in explaining the psychological *meaning* of physical symptoms, it proved unable to clarify the physical *mechanisms* that would account for a particular psychological issue leading to specific physical and pathological processes.

This dilemma began with Freud himself, who refused to confront the psychosomatic problem, and side-stepped it—except in his famous study of symptom formation in hysteria—in such a way as to situate psychoanalysis squarely on the psychic side of the bodymind continuum. Orthodox analysts since Freud would view somatic processes as a language of the body to be interpreted psychologically, thereby ignoring completely the body itself and its dynamics. This explains why many psychotherapists interested in the psychosomatic question took their lead from a physician specializing in physical medicine, Georg Groddeck, a contemporary of Freud, who chose to work with the psychosomatic problem directly, beginning with the physical body and its complex manifestations. Unlike Freud, Groddeck did not believe that an understanding of the meaning of illness could be divorced from an intimate knowledge of the body.

As we review the classic psychoanalytic studies of psychosomatics in the following pages, then, the reader should bear in mind that we do this in order to better understand the symbolism of the psyche and the importance of grasping the meaning of physical symptoms. It will become evident that psychoanalysis itself is not sufficient in the treatment of psychosomatic disorders, which is why modern behavioral medicine has all but supplanted psychoanalysis as the treatment of choice in such disorders. We include this survey of analytic attempts to understand the bodymind and its interactions in order to revive a philosophical rigor that is totally absent from modern behavioral medicine. While the former might justifiably be termed pure philosophy, the latter only appears to be a pure science. Both approaches, it will be argued, suffer from a rigid stance—psychological in the first case and physiological in the second—that fails to appreciate the fundamental dynamics of the bodymind.

The hypothesis of this chapter is that Western concepts of psychosomatics must be situated in the larger context of bodymind energetics. Energetics, as inherent in acupuncture theory and practice, encompasses psychological and physiological events, placing acupuncture in the realm of behavioral medicine and at the same time widening the philosophical position of behavioral medicine to incorporate energetic phenomena. This reformulation of behavioral medicine as *energetic* may well lead, in the decades to come, to a restructuring of medicine and psychiatry around behavioral, energetic, dynamic vectors. This was the vision of the pioneers of psychosomatic medicine, whose work must not be ignored.

Early in his career Freud attempted to solve the "psychosomatic problem" in his treatment of hysterics, only to admit in a letter to his colleague Fleiss that while he was not content to promote his psychological theory without an organic basis, he had no theoretical or therapeutic solution to the psychosomatic problem and thus would have to act as if *only the psychological lay before him.*[13] Freud and his followers hoped for a day when endocrinology and physiology would be able to explain the somatic basis for the psychic processes they discovered. This wish was never fulfilled, as we shall see, and it is for this reason that acupuncture-energetic physiology, which is consistent with psychosomatic concepts of psychoenergetic functioning, will prove most valuable.

Freud skirted the philosophical issues involved in the psychosomatic problem, deeming psychoanalysis unsuitable for an exploration or treatment of the somatic component of most psychological complaints. He did not seek *"to explain* the connection and interaction of psyche and soma so much as to *understand* what the patient experiences in the interaction with the therapist, how he behaved, and what function the psychosomatic symptomatic behavior had in *this* connection."[14]

According to this position, the only physical symptom accessible to psychoanalytic treatment was hysteria. In his major contribution to psychosomatic theory, Freud explained that in a hysterical *conversion reaction* the physical symptom, such as loss of sight or paralysis, was not a physiological event but rather a *representation* of one or several unacceptable thoughts grounded in infantile sexuality.[15]

In the hysterical conversion reaction, then, the physical symptom was a representation of a specific psychological conflict or issue and the conversion process a form of psychological repression. Once the patient was brought to an understanding of the psychic core of his complaint, the somatic basis and symptomatology dissolved.

This was not the case, Freud thought, with most of the physical components of other emotional or psychological states. The physical symptoms of an anxiety attack—including, for example, increased perspiration, altered cardiac activity and breathing, muscle twitches and spasms, increased hunger, diarrhea, loss of sensation, dizziness and the like—were, according to Freud, concomitant with and *equivalent to the anxiety attack,* and could even replace the anxiety attack itself. These symptoms could not be broken down further by psychoanalytic interpretation or technique for the simple reason that they signified nothing more than the body's natural reaction to fear and stress—that is, a physiological event with no psychological meaning to uncover. This is why Freud believed that such problems could not be treated by psychotherapy.[16]

In the "equivalent of an anxiety attack," then, the physical symptom is not a representation of a psychic conflict but rather is the result of a "somatic excitation [that] is actually denied access to the psychic and is abreacted in the formation of an organic symptom."[17] In the formation of the physical symptoms that accompany anxiety, Freud maintained, no psychic activity occurs, so that the physical symptoms exist alongside the anxiety rather than representing some repressed psychological conflict. While hysterical conversion symptoms are related to psychological *repression,* somatic anxiety symptoms are related to somatic *projection.*

The technique of free association in psychoanalysis enabled the therapist to decipher the symbolic message of the conversion symptoms, but because anxiety equivalence symptoms were thought not to represent psychic ideas, this technique was not applicable to them.

Psychoanalysts focusing on the psychosomatic problem after Freud have attempted to resolve the issue of "conversion" versus "equivalence" in several ways, as we shall see.

The Body Speaks

Pioneers of classic psychosomatics were able to take up where Freud left off by recognizing that there was a *body language* inherent in anxiety equivalence that was indeed amenable to psychotherapeutic investigation and treatment.

Analysts such as Paul Federn, Felix Deutsch, and Franz Alexander went far in developing an understanding of this body language, by shifting the focus of investigation away from the psychological meaning of the symptoms and toward the psychoenergetic nature of the functional disturbance itself. Instead of focusing on the underlying meaning of an organic symptom, these therapists concerned themselves with *how* the body and the physical symptom communicate. In discussing a case of asthma, Federn explained the symptom of asthma as a fixation of psychic energy in the respiratory system itself, including the olfactory zone. Referring to this case, Freud diagnosed it as a "fixation hysteria" whereby compliance in the physical body predisposes a particular organ system to dysfunction resulting in the development of somatic symptoms.[18]

At about the same time, in 1917, Georg Groddeck criticized Freud's view of psychosomatics. He did not agree that the hysteric was the only one who could induce physical illness for identifiable, unconscious reasons. He believed that everyone somatized psychic conflicts far more often than Freud assumed. Groddeck believed the psychic force at the root of life, which he termed the *It*, found symbolic expression through physical as well as psychological means. He thought that somatic symptoms in physical illness protected the person's *It* (Life Force) against noxious stimuli. In speaking of common physical symptoms in respiratory disorders (coughing up of thick phlegm and so on), Groddeck wrote, "whatever, despite the It's ability to close off entry to the individual's inner being, does penetrate and appear poisonous to the It, is dissolved and swathed in slime, cast out and spat upon afterward. . . . The extraordinary thing about this process is that *the unconscious equates physical and psychic invaders and treats them in the same way.*"[19]

As we have seen, this is true in acupuncture-energetic theory as well.

When a person reacts on a somatic-energetic level, developing meridian disturbances and resultant physical symptoms, it is both to fend off external environmental stress and to divert and absorb internal emotional stress in order to maintain bodymind integrity. In both the acupuncture perspective and Groddeck's formulation, the body is a protector of the psyche, capable of functioning as defensive barrier and shock absorber.

The Body Complies

Felix Deutsch, a Viennese physician and analyst, went beyond Freud's theories by postulating that conversion processes occurred throughout life, not only in the neurotic but in the healthy individual as well. He observed conversion processes in functional and organic disorders and concluded that the process was a lifelong means of discharging and preventing accumulations of psychic energy. He felt that modern society forced people to suppress psychic drives and desires, leading to an accumulation of this energy. Thus, the ongoing conversion process, which he termed "conversion stream," was necessary as a reaction pattern for the general maintenance of health.[20]

Deutsch labeled such common conversion processes as blushing, nervous headache, or nervous sweating the "language of the organic," facilitating "the discharge of pent-up libido, of affect debris, which burdens the unconscious through its accumulation."[21] Functional or organic disorders develop when there occurs an inhibited overinvestment of repressed psychic energy in an organ-functional system. The specific organ system affected is determined by what Deutsch termed "somatic compliance." This somatic compliance, also termed "organ inferiority" by Alfred Adler, could arise from a constitutional weakness or from an organic injury early in life affecting the formation of the body-ego and one's psychological way of viewing the body. The result would be inappropriate or deficient psychoenergetic defenses that predispose a specific organ system to accumulation of psychic energy. In this sense, the weakened organ functional system serves as a safety valve for the discharge of potentially noxious psychic energy. Interestingly, Deutsch noted that this "somatic compliance," this *readiness for illness*, might occur out of an unconscious identification with a "significant other" suffering from a complaint in the same organ system.[22]

A child may learn to discharge psychic accumulation through conversion of this pent-up energy into the vascular system, for example, generating a migraine headache or a stomach-ache, patterning such behavior on that observed in significant others in the family.

Deutsch's concept of body language as a constant conversion process is a major contribution to the development of a psychosomatic theory. This idea is remarkably similar to the acupuncture concept of invasion of internal and external pathogenic factors that are warded off by the somatic-energetic meridian systems.[23]

Body Neuroses

Franz Alexander, like Freud and unlike Deutsch, maintained the fundamental distinction between conversion processes and the organic psychosomatic disorders, which he termed organ "vegetative" neuroses. While the conversion symptom was an *expression* or a *representation* of an emotional or psychic conflict, the vegetative or organ neurosis was the reaction of a specific organ-functional system to unabated or regularly occurring psychic and emotional states.[24] In other words, functional disturbances (organ neuroses), in which analysis of the tissue showed no morphological change but only a disturbance in the "coordination and the intensity of its function," were seen as distinct from conversion reactions, which were merely representations.[25]

"A vegetative neurosis is not an attempt to express an emotion but is a physiological response of the vegetative organ to constant or to periodically returning emotional states. Elevation of blood pressure, for example, under the influence of rage, does not relieve the rage but is a physiological component in the phenomenon of rage."[26]

This is not very different from Deutsch's concept of constant conversion processes, for in both cases specific organ-functional reaction patterns are activated by accompanying psychoenergetic defenses. Interestingly, "vegetative neuroses" are precisely what the Chinese classical medical textbooks discuss in great detail, though in different form, when they speak of "organ patterns of disharmony."

An important aspect of Alexander's work was its grounding in physiology and its discussion of the basic reaction patterns of the autonomic nervous system, namely, sympathetic and parasympathetic reactions. Also crucial in Alexander's view was the realization, still virtually unacknowledged by allopathic medicine, that a sustained functional complaint exists prior to most physical change and organic disease, as Deutsch and Groddeck had already demonstrated.

Classic Psychosomatics

Orthodox medicine defined a psychosomatic disorder as one in which the predominant etiological factor in the disease was psychological in origin. Alexander rejected this point of view, stating that available evidence "points to multi-causal explanations in all branches of medicine."[27] He maintained that a purely psychogenic explanation for a psychosomatic disease, such as peptic ulcer, was not sufficient to explain the disorder. "Local or general somatic factors, as yet ill-defined, must be assumed, and only the co-existence of both kinds of factors, emotional and somatic, can account for this formation."[28] It is here that acupuncture energetics will prove of special interest to psychotherapists, as the apparently "ill-defined local or general somatic factors" are in fact well delineated in the patterns of acupuncture, and have been observed and verified over and over again for more than two thousand years.

The relative importance of emotional factors, as compared with somatic factors, varies greatly from one individual to another, depending on that person's location on the bodymind continuum. This being the case, Alexander concluded that a specific diagnostic category of "psychosomatic disease" was unthinkable. "Theoretically," he concludes, "every disease is psychosomatic since emotional factors influence all body processes through nervous and humoral pathways."[29]

Psychosomatic medicine, as understood and developed by Alexander, added four major factors to the discussion of the etiology of disease: the nature of infant care (breast feeding, weaning, toilet training), traumatic emotional accidents in infancy and childhood, the emotional climate of the family and the personalities of the significant others in the family, and later emotional experiences in intimate interpersonal relations.[30] These factors are almost totally ignored in orthodox Western as well as traditional Chinese medicine but must be incorporated in any sensible Western practice of bodymind integration to fill a void noted by early analysts, namely, to define the physiological dynamics inherent in the genesis of psychosomatic disorders.

Body Reactions

The organ function reacts in one of two ways to an emotional disturbance or perceived threat. Either the sympathetic system becomes activated in preparation for "fight or flight," or else the parasympathetic system prepares for introverted withdrawal from external activity to allow the organism to "rest and digest" and attend to internal demands.

"The sympathetic nervous system is involved in the preparation of the organism for fight or flight by modifying the vegetative processes in a way most useful in emergency situations."[31] In this process, it inhibits anabolic, parasympathetic processes, thereby acting as a natural "inhibitor of gastrointestinal activity."[32] Through sympathetic function, the heart drives the distribution of blood to the exterior musculature, the lungs, and the cerebrum. Thus, the blood pressure rises, carbohydrates are mobilized out of storage, and the adrenals are stimulated.

The parasympathetic functions, on the other hand, lead to an introversion of energy as the individual withdraws into vegetative existence, allowing for relaxation, growth, and maintenance of the organism. The parasympathetic influences lead to stimulation of gastrointestinal activity and storing of sugar in the liver.[33]

Disturbances of a *sympathetic nature* result, Alexander maintains, from "inhibition or repression of self-assertive, hostile impulses," where this inhibition results in the absence of actual fight or flight. The organism and the self are in a chronic state of readiness for outwardly directed activity, a state accompanied by all the corresponding sympathetic system physiological reactions (increased heart rate, high blood pressure, dilation of peripheral blood vessels, stepped-up metabolism).[34] Some of the disorders that occur if sympathetic activation is prolonged, or a person is especially vulnerable to sympathetic stimuli, are cardiac neuroses, migraines, hypertension, hyperthyroidism, and rheumatoid arthritis.

In *parasympathetic* reactions, on the other hand, the bodymind reacts by withdrawing from action into a dependent state. This type of reaction, termed "vegetative retreat" by Alexander, is like running into the arms of the mother and falling asleep there.[35] A person who reacts in this way does not marshall defenses to ward off external danger but rather retreats from the danger and looks for help. This dependent desire for security and help is associated with the desire to be fed and thus produces increased gastric activity. The functional disorders of the gastrointestinal tract belong here, as do bronchial asthma, fatigue states, and such disorders as peptic ulcer, constipation, diarrhea, and colitis. A predisposition toward either sympathetic or parasympathetic reaction patterns develops as a result of a multiplicity of factors, including external stimuli and the somatic and psychoenergetic reaction patterns learned in early childhood when the infant is totally dependent upon the mother for nourishment and protection. These two reaction patterns may be viewed as the two basic prototypes for all somatic reaction patterns, with one directed toward the outside world and the other directed inward.

If we superimpose Alexander's sympathetic and parasympathetic reaction patterns on the Five-Phase energetic physiology chart presented in Chapter 2, where the deficient Yin Root was seen to lead to Yang (sympathetic) reaction patterns and the deficient Yang Root to lead to Yin (parasympathetic) reaction patterns, an extremely use-

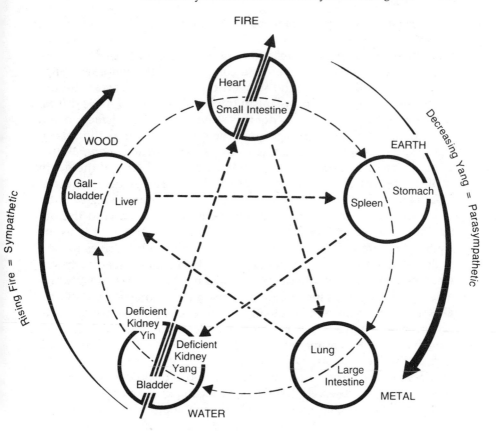

ful framework emerges, not only for categorizing psychosomatic reaction patterns but also for predicting predispositions to disease.

The Body Self and the Drives

The concept of *body ego* developed by Freud is at the root of the bodymind problem. He said the "ego is ultimately derived from bodily sensations, chiefly from those springing from the surface of the body. It may thus be regarded as a mental projection of the surface of the body, besides . . . representing the superficies of the mental apparatus."[36]

Fenichel, an analyst working in the psychosomatic field, took this concept one step further when he described the development of the "body image" as the core of the ego. The formation of a psychic representation of the body and its organ functions makes it possible to develop an image of one's ego. The body self precedes the psychic self; or rather, the psychological self is fundamentally physical in origin.

Another specialist in psychosomatic medicine, Schilder, saw the body image or "body scheme" as a complex psychic configuration.[37] Disagreeing with Freud, who viewed the psychic drives as the dynamic force propelling the organism toward *satisfaction* of these drives, Schilder thought the key was not this striving toward satisfaction and relaxation, but the striving "toward the *object* that brings the relaxation," and he saw this process as primarily a constructive one. "Thus I am opposed," stated Schilder," to the Freudian theory of the death instinct and the repetition compulsion. I now recognize as the ego instinct only those trends of taking, holding, and possessing that follow entirely the general rules of instinctivity, strive toward the object, and revive themselves in a new ardor on new objects."[38] It seems equally important, however, to take into account other drives having to do with a refusal to hold, to work, or to be arranged in any particular system at all. While these drives need not be seen as constituting a death instinct, as Freud finally conceived them, they do constitute, as is stated by Deleuze and Guattari (authors of a provocative study of psychoenergetics), a fundamental pole of psychic functioning, namely, the pole that moves toward disorganization and entropy as part of the life process.[39]

In developing a psychosomatic concept of skin disorders, Max Schur, a psychoanalyst, observed that the ego functioned as an organ of adaptation utilizing psychic energy that had been neutralized. He thought that this neutralization of psychic energy took place through the progressive "desomatization of behavior." In early childhood, the child reacts to anxiety-producing situations by means of uncoordinated bodily movements affecting the entire body (primary process behavior). As the central nervous system and the psyche mature, the primary process behavior of somatization of the drives is progressively replaced by secondary process behavior, namely, thinking, and with a withdrawal of psychic energy away from the soma (desomatization). "Thinking increasingly replaces the diffuse vegetative and motor discharge reactions."[40] If the maturing ego can work through anxiety as well as respond to it, its actions will be desomatized and there will be no physical manifestations of excitation discharge. A *resomatization*, on the other hand, can be understood, in this view, as an ego "regression" to primary process behavior. The predisposition to somatize is due to constitutional as well as developmental factors related to the ways, both physical and psychological, in which one copes with the outside world. Schur, like Deutsch, maintained the existence of a strict correlation between a *specific emotional state* and a *somatic reaction state*, which "denotes a readiness to react somatically."[41] Ammon expanded on this concept, seeing the psychosomatic symptom as an ultimately self-destructive attempt to fill out and compensate for an ego deficit that evolved during the constitution of the body ego and its boundary, and thus as an attempt to preserve the integrity of the person.[42] He referred to this ego deficit as a "hole in the ego."

The Primal Embrace

The ego develops, according to Schur, within the world of what Spitz, a psychiatrist, termed the "primal cavity" created by the cradling arms of the mother as well as the oral cavity of the infant's mouth as it takes in the breast.[43] This world of the primal cavity, where the mother opens her arms to *give* totally to the child by *taking in* the child, and the child opens its mouth *to receive* by *incorporating* the mother's breast, serves as the experiential field where the infant develops its basic ego functions and the sense of boundaries that allows it to separate internal and external reality. The parameters of this experiential field are constituted by the mother's arms, her breast, the skin of mother and child, the infant's mouth, and so on. Deleuze and Guattari talk of the emerging ego extending outward toward new objects, beginning with the mother's breast, as *attraction,* and of the undifferentiated force field of the primal cavity as *repulsion.* They see those two primary forces, attraction and repulsion, as the fundamental poles of the life force (*It*) itself. They term the forces of attraction "desiring-machines," forces that cause the ego to strive toward objects with which it can forge a working connection. They term the forces of repulsion the "body-without-organs", which refers to the primal embrace with the mother, that frees the infant from the attracting objects and allows it to return to an undifferentiated state, prior to the organization of the body ego or the self (entropy as part of the process of life). The desiring-machines propel the ego, as in Schilder's view, toward new objects and connections. The body-without-organs, on the other hand, is a way of depicting that aspect of psychoenergetic dynamics that tends toward disintegration and breakdown. In the view of Deleuze and Guattari, this apparently destructive, nonproductive part of the life process, this "anti-production," is an essential part of psychic functioning: "Everything stops dead for a moment, everything freezes in place—and then the whole process will begin all over again. From a certain point of view, it would be much better if nothing worked, if nothing functioned, never being born, escaping the wheel of continual birth and rebirth, no mouth to suck with, no anus to shit through. Will the machines run so badly, their component pieces fall apart to such a point, that they will return to nothingness, and thus allow us to return to nothingness . . . . Desiring machines make us an organism; but at the very heart of this production, the body suffers from being organized in this way, from not having some other sort of organization, or no organization at all."[44]

The concept of the body-without-organs is a way of conceptualizing the process of psychosomatic dysfunction as part of the bodymind-energetic dynamic itself.

The shift from an excited state of desiring-production to one of exhaustion and breakdown is most readily observable in the behavior of the very young child. The child may become attracted to any object that crosses its path, examining it visually and manually, and eventually putting it into its mouth. It becomes one with this object, internalizing both the object itself and its reactions to the object. This momentary discovery of surfaces and boundaries, both internal and external, will help form the child's body ego. Yet at the same time the excited state will inevitably shift into one of overstimulation and fatigue. The child will have no choice but to let go of all objects, all desiring-production, and sink into the warm, dark, protective, womb-like cavity created by the mother's embrace. It will nurse itself either back to an active state or into a deep, uterine-like sleep. This breakdown is often accompanied by tears or tantrums as the body suffers from its attempts to organize itself and the outside world. When such momentary psychological breakdowns are properly integrated, thanks to adequate responses on the mother's part, they simply become part of the maturing body image and ego structure. In pathological development, on the other hand, in which the mother or other caretaker is not able to help the child integrate these temporary breakdowns, the process of psychosomatic disintegration may become an end in itself.

According to most modern psychosomatic researchers, the essential factor in avoiding serious psychosomatic disorders is "adequate mothering," a concept developed by Winnicott, a British pediatrician and psychoanalyst.

The development of body functions and different modes of reacting to the environment are based upon a positive, affective, physical interaction between the mother and child, "during the course of which the child introjects the mother's attitude and behavior toward him and thus develops a body ego which allows an initial differentiation between the internal and external world with the help of the earliest ego boundary, namely the body ego boundary."[45]

Since the 1960s, research in ego psychology and object relations has focused heavily on the role of the mother in the development of her child's ego boundary. In this view, the child's boundary will be "that much stronger and more flexible, the more capable the mother is of experiencing the child's needs, the more she is in a positive position to understand and respond to the child's preverbal body language as being meaningful and important."[46] This holds true not only for post-natal development but for prenatal development as well.

Ammon, in his concept of a hole in the ego, maintains that the early ego, faced with repeated failure by the mother (inadequate mothering) as well as lack on the part of the primary family group to pay sufficient or consistent attention, experiences an *existential abandonment anxiety*, which is filled up to a certain extent by the symptom.[47] The truly psychosomatic child of a "psychosomatically-inducing mother" will overadapt to external demands by a meaningless mechanistic functioning and will react "to every demand regarding the active determination of his own identity with a flight into the false identity of the psychosomatic. In place of the question, 'who am I?' which is combined with existential anxiety for the patient, comes the question, 'what do I have?' for which he constantly seeks an answer. In other words, the question of one's own identity is replaced by a question of the symptom, which functions as a substitute identity."[48]

The symptom therefore harkens back to the internalized mother of early childhood, who would react to the child's attempts at active demarcation of Self by paying loving attention only when the child was sick. Here the symptom replaces or constitutes the sense of identity.

Psychosomatic Reaction Patterns

While Ammon's work was directed toward overtly pathological psychosomatic disorders, based on inadequate mothering in a psychosomatizing familial community, Deleuze and Guattari's view of psychosomatic energetic functioning takes into account, as already stated, a built-in process of breakdown in the relatively normal child as well. In their view, psychosomatic symptoms are a manifestation of the functional move toward disorganization and an undifferentiated state from which new organizations are possible and to which we always return. The body-without-organs is the surface created by the primal embrace with the mother, which itself echoes prenatal potentiality and the return to an undifferentiated state.

In essence, what the psychosomatic perspective teaches us is that somatic symptoms are anything but simple manifestations of physiological functioning, and that they are therefore often (if not always) bound up with a complex web of experiences in which the developing self and the outside world are at odds with each other, and the bodymind reacts to these conflicts as to an external stress *by somatic as well as psychic reaction patterns.*

Reconstructing Inner Worlds

Whereas classic psychosomatics went far in describing bodymind interactions, it often proved therapeutically inadequate in the treatment of psychosomatic disorders. Doubtless this is due, in large part, to the nature of the psychoanalytic process itself, which often works far too slowly to resolve the somatic component of a psychosomatic complaint. Rather than grounding a person in the bodymind as it exists in the world, psychoanalysis tends to reduce the living psychosomatic reaction patterns to static, intellectualized psychosexual constructs. While analytic interpretation may help a person understand the meaning of his bodymind imbalance, it rarely suffices to significantly alter the complaint itself.

In the first half of this century, new psychotherapeutic schools were being formed by those who chose to diverge from the orthodox psychoanalytic framework and who sought new theories and new therapeutics to make up for clearly perceived shortcomings of the orthodox approach.

One approach was to become known as phenomenological or existential psychology.[49]

Confronted with the atrocities of fascism, and at a loss to explain the psychodynamic forces at work in such a collective madness, a significant number of European psychiatrists and analysts inspired by Nietzsche began to examine human nature and the role of psychotherapy in the modern era.

They criticized the orthodox psychoanalytic approach, suggesting that the analyst rarely perceived or knew the patient as he or she really was, but rather as a projection of the therapist's own analytical theories.

Instead of viewing psychological abnormalities as deviations from some preconceived psychological norm, these phenomenological psychotherapists viewed such crises as modifications in the patient's own structure of *being-in-the-world.* Basing their views on Heidegger's phenomenological analysis of existence, itself inspired by Nietzsche's probing analyses at the turn of the century, these therapists sought to understand phenomena in the patient's life not from some safe, objective, theoretical vantage point, but rather from within the *subjective* world of the patient as he or she experienced it.

The phenomenological approach attempted to establish, not a new school of psychotherapy, but a sufficiently broad philosophical groundwork for the study of the very structure of human existence, regardless of the psychotherapeutic approach.

Unimpressed by the attempts of European psychiatry and psychology to define themselves as science rather than philosophy, the phenomenologists believed that the most purely scientific of pursuits, as was later articulated by modern physicists from Einstein on, was rooted in a rigorous philosophical investigation of one's own being-in-the-universe.

One of the major ideas in the air at the turn of the century, brought starkly into focus by the fascist movement, was the problematic nature of humanity alienated from itself.

No one confronted the issues of the human existential dilemma more forcefully than Nietzsche. Even Freud, who claimed to have renounced his attempt to read Nietzsche's dense work, was obliged to admit, in a statement that foreshadowed the discovery of the psychoanalytic method, that "Nietzsche had a more penetrating knowledge of himself than any other man who ever lived or was ever likely to live."[50]

Opposed to all ideologies and dogma that enslaved human beings, Nietzsche proclaimed the need for a new philosopher who would confront every truth directly, in his own personal experience, to see if an idea could be "lived with" on a personal level. Setting the stage for the later phenomenological and existential thinkers, he proclaimed, "we others who thirst for reason want to look our experiences in the eye as severely as at a scientific experiment . . . ! We ourselves want to be our own experiment and guinea-pigs!"[51]

Nietzsche's formulation of the underlying force in human beings, which he termed "will to power," had nothing to do, as some erroneously concluded, with a desire for power, but rather referred to the will to be fully alive, to experience one's full potential, to do whatever one did with one's energy raised to the nth power. In the affirmation of one's own being, in its basest as well as its highest elements, a person creates his own values and gives birth to his true essence.

This was carried over into phenomenological and existential psychotherapy, in which the therapist was viewed not as a medical scientist focused on mental disease, but rather as a philosopher-guide and co-explorer focused on the patient's own deeply felt experience of the bodymind. The role of the therapist, in helping the patient resolve emotional blocks and overcome psychological barriers, was thus conceived as a confrontation on the part of the patient with the fundamental freedom to change by realizing untapped potential.

From this perspective, *anxiety* denotes the presence of a potential for being different, for changing, before the change has occurred. Confronted in therapy with the issue of fulfilling his or her potential, a patient develops a deep sense of anxiety, as Rollo May, a prominent American existential psychotherapist, points out,[52] and if the patient denies or fails to realize this potential, the result will be a sense of "philosophical, ontological guilt." This sense of guilt, entirely distinct from the psychoanalytic guilt stemming from violation of a parental prohibition (neurotic guilt feeling), is a natural guilt, a *being-indebted-to-oneself*.

Whereas the guilt discovered in psychoanalysis can become very removed from oneself, and dissolved by psychoanalytic interpretation, as it is absolved in the confession box by the priest's words, the phenomenologist would maintain that existential guilt goes to the core of one's being, as it confronts one with all that could have been done but never was.[53]

Another aspect of this existential guilt is a guilt toward others for not perceiving them as fully separate beings-in-the-world in their own right. Realization of these two forms of guilt or indebtedness, as well as a more spiritual guilt for existing separate from the forces of the cosmos and indebtedness to the cosmos for our own existence, serve as dynamic catalysts, in the phenomenological therapeutic process, for confronting us with our capacities to transform ourselves.

While the phenomenological approach offers no specific techniques, it does afford therapists of all persuasions with a philosophical approach revolving around three methods for situating the patient's inner experiences and reconstructing the state of being-in-the-world from within.

These three main methods utilized by the early phenomenological therapists to investigate the patient's inner universe, as presented by the phenomenological psychiatrist Henri Ellenberger, are *descriptive phenomenology, genetic-structural phenomenology,* and *categorical analysis*.[54]

In *descriptive phenomenology,* the therapist constructs a detailed subjective description—from the patient's point of view—of the patient's experiences in an effort to empathize as fully as possible with these experiences. Carl Rogers's well-known "client-centered psychotherapy," wherein the therapist serves as a mirror to reflect the patient's processes of becoming back to him or her for clarification, could be termed an example of the descriptive phenomenological approach.

By means of the *genetic-structural method,* the phenomenological therapist attempts to find the underlying "genetic" or constitutional factors that, once grasped, would enable the patient and therapist to reconstruct the entire gestalt of the individual's current state of being. This method postulates a fundamental unity among the different events in a person's life, with an eye toward understanding the effects on this lived life of the underlying constitutional forces.

The third method, the *categorical analytic method,* works by taking a set of phenomenological coordinates—space, time, causality, materiality—and analyzing how the patient experiences each of these coordinates. This is done in order to reconstruct the patient's inner experienced universe of being. In this aspect of the phenomenological approach, the therapist works to situate the ways in which the patient experiences his or her own temporality, the speed and duration and tempo of life, and experiences of the ebb and flow of *time;* the patient's relationship to *space,* to up and down, to right and left— the reference point for spatial awareness being the space of one's own body, including the different "spaces" created by the experience of the senses. Hence, the phenomenologist postulates an experience of tactile space, visual space, auditory space, olfactory space, and the like. Acupuncture therapy is especially useful in helping the patient experience the spaces of the body and the ways in which bodily forces become trapped in specific areas of the body.

The next phase in categorical analysis is to lead the patient to explore his or her causality, to determine whether he or she lives life as predetermined by some prior set of dictates, as due to randomness and chance, or as the result of the intentionality of the individual who affirms past choices and the capacity to make new ones. Finally, the phenomenological approach helps a person experience the materiality of the world itself (its fluidity, its softness, its hardness, its heat and cold, its light and darkness, and so forth), especially with respect to the four elements of nature: fire, earth, water, and air. While the phenomenologists have developed some fascinating descriptions of the experience of these four elements in the psychotherapeutic process, the Five Element tradition of acupuncture as previously discussed entails an ongoing, in-depth exploration of the patient's inner experiences of these material elements as they affect his or her own being-in-the-world.

Whichever of these three methods is utilized, Ellenberger concludes, "the aim of the investigation is the *reconstruction of the inner world of experience of the subject.* Each individual has his own way of experiencing temporality, spatiality, causation, materiality, but each of these coordinates must be understood in relation to the others and to the total 'world.' "[55]

The importance of the phenomenological approach as it relates to the psychosomatic question we have been addressing is that it obliges the therapist to focus on the reality of existence *as experienced and expressed by the patient,* in all of its physical, psychological, and spiritual dimensions. It is especially useful as a philosophical orientation for the bodymind-energetic approach, as it situates the therapeutic process in the patient's own lived experience, and all analyses stem from these actual experiences rather than from a preconceived therapeutic and interpretative grid, as is the case with psychoanalysis. In this sense it helps ground the encounter between therapist and client in the here-and-now of the person's *presence* and *present*, and works to reconstruct as fully as possible the person's inner world, both physical and mental, in order for the person to become more aware of his or her potential for growth and change.

Acupuncture energetics provides the basis for an investigation of the dynamics of the body process; classic psychosomatics serves as a point of departure for investigating psychoenergetic functioning. The phenomenological approach yields a philosophical stance toward therapeutic work, consistent with acupuncture therapy and psychosomatics, that unifies somatic and psychoenergetic formulations in the subjective realm of the person's own being-in-the-world.

The preceding summary of classic psychosomatics and phenomenological psychology is meant to provide body workers, acupuncture therapists, and psychotherapists with a solid basis for understanding psychosomatic interactions. In Part II of this book, we shall begin to sketch a phenomenology of the bodymind-energetic systems through a combined perspective drawing on the psychosomatic- and acupuncture-energetic points of view and informed by the phenomenological philosophical orientation.

We shall conclude this chapter with a brief look at modern psychosomatics, especially as it has developed out of research on *stress.*

THE STRESS CONNECTION

While the classic psychosomatic and phenomenological perspectives have yielded great insights into bodymind interactions, modern behavioral psychological research, especially in the United States, has tended to be far less philosophical and more pragmatic. This behavioral approach has been especially important in its understanding of the "stress connection" in modern life, as a major precipitating factor in the genesis of body/mind splits of various sorts.

A modern behavioral approach to psychosomatics developed out of the psychophysiological investigation of stress. These research findings are less theoretically dense than their European classic psychosomatic and phenomenological predecessors, but are of great therapeutic significance. In any case, one needs a combination of philosophy and science, of poetry and pragmatism, to promote healing as well as to fully appreciate the complexity of bodymind functioning.

Kenneth Pelletier offers a perspective on psychosomatic disorders drawn from research, literature, and practice involving the psychophysiology and treatment of stress and its disorders. He identifies major triggers of stress in environmental factors, such as noise and air pollution, overcrowding, high-pressure jobs, and constant competition. Other severe stressors may be financial pressures, family quarrels, the death of a loved one, difficulties with one's boss or co-workers, and the like. Less obvious sources are the reactions to those sources of stress themselves, leading to what Pelletier terms "a free-floating anxiety" and to "inexplicable variations in sleeping or eating patterns, muscle tension or spasms, and numerous other disturbing symptoms."[56] These types of disorders and disturbing symptoms are among those that commonly bring people to acupuncture therapists for treatment.

Of course, not all stress is harmful. Any event—marriage, a desired pregnancy, a job promotion, or even a vacation—that obliges us to adapt and change causes stress that leads to changes in psychological and physiological adaptation patterns. Stress that is short-lived, or whose source is easily identified, exists as a sort of challenge to the organism to adapt and move on. "However, when the sources of stress are multiple, unclear, or chronic, then the individual does not return to normal physiological functioning as readily."[57] This can lead either to a severe stress reaction or to an unabated stress reaction that slowly wears away at the psychosomatic complex.

Psychosocial stress has become a dangerous and growing source of psychological and physiological disorders in our fast-paced culture. The foremost illnesses of modern society, cardiovascular disease, cancer, arthritis, and respiratory diseases, are due in large part to increased psychosocial stress as well as to denatured food and a contaminated environment. As Pelletier notes, fifty to eighty percent of all diseases can be attributed to psychosomatic or stress-related factors. Common disorders such as hypertension; hyperthyroidism; migraine and tension headaches; sleep-onset insomnia; alcoholism and drug addiction; peptic ulcer; different forms of colitis; asthma; many forms of dermatitis and hives; hay fever; arthritis; circulatory disorders such as Raynaud's disease, amenorrhea, and premenstrual syndrome; and cardiac functional disorders such as palpitations and rapid heart beat are classified even by orthodox medicine as psychosomatic.[58]

If this is indeed the case, then mental health practitioners must begin shifting their focus away from treatment of disease or correction of pathological conditions to stress reduction and prevention of disease through concerted programs in health maintenance. The holistic approach suggested by Pelletier focuses on the whole person and sees any disorder as a complex interplay of societal, physiological, and psychological factors; the personality configuration of the individual; and his or her capacity and methods for coping with these factors.

Insight-oriented approaches to psychological stress disorders can be quite helpful, but insight into the development of a psychosomatic disorder will not necessarily help correct the disorder. In addition to insight or awareness into the source of stress, the behavior pattern associated with the stress, and its significance to the individual's life, it must be "explained to the psychosomatic patient [that there is] a connection between behavior, attitudes and the autonomic neurophysiological functions. People need to understand and sense this connection before they can learn specific skills to help them alleviate stress."[59]

Psychotherapeutic approaches are strong in insight and meaning, but weak in understanding the specific somatic factors involved and consequently often therapeutically ineffective in modifying dysfunctional somatic patterns. Perhaps this is why there are a few remarkable cases to be found in the psychoanalytic psychosomatic literature in which major psychosomatic complaints such as hysterical paralysis have been cured, while at the same time there is little reported sustained success with complaints like migraine, colitis, asthma, heart palpitations, and the everyday psychosomatic complaints of many patients. In all fairness, a psychoanalyst may not elect to focus on alleviating these somatic symptoms. Nevertheless, if migraine headache is taken to be the result of a particular personality configuration reacting to unabated stress in a consistent fashion, then we cannot be satisfied merely with the understanding that the headache is a symbol of repressed rage. For the dysfunction in the head and neck vessels, and the tightness of the musculature, are energetically depleting states that can prove quite injurious over time. Paradoxically, then, those who choose to focus on the deepest, most spiritual level of a person's being, by ignoring the somatic dynamics, may end up not only providing a less effective therapy for relieving specific psychosomatic symptoms and complaints, but actually contributing to the development of psychosomatic disorders.

It is common in long-term psychotherapy for a patient to achieve insight and feel far better in the self, while at the same time developing vague pains or an annoying complaint of a psychosomatic nature. We believe this is because achievement of insight bypasses the somatic energetic systems, which must be palpated and treated locally. For if one bypasses the somatic systems, a psychosomatic reaction pattern may become fixed in a predisposed or "compliant" organ functional system, setting the stage for some future physical complaint. The intensification of energy accumulation in a somatic zone, as we know from acupuncture energetics, leads to a blockage in the circulation of vital fluids and energy, resulting in such "stagnant" conditions as lumps, cysts, tumors, and the like. The goal of acupuncture energetics is to open up the way for a free circulation of these vital elements and thus to more adaptive responses on the part of the individual.

Pelletier advocates the combined use of *insight*, to help a person understand the meaning of the symptoms, and *education*, to teach the person the relationship between attitude, behavior, and the reactions of the sympathetic and parasympathetic systems. For a change to occur in body image and body function, a person needs to "sense" the interconnection of all of these factors, and our primitive and primary mode of sensing such things is in and through the body. Acupuncture somatic-energetic theory and therapy, when conceived as a bodymind-energetic approach, is an excellent vehicle for integrating insight, education, and a bodily felt sense of improved function for the client. This same approach has been advocated by certain psychotherapists trained in body work, such as Reichians, but these approaches lack a sufficiently elaborated somatic-energetic theory for understanding the complexity of most psychosomatic complaints.

Proponents of biofeedback, such as Pelletier, emphasize the healing potential of this therapy in teaching a person to recognize and thereby gain control over bodymind-dysfunctional patterns. In like fashion, one could conceive of acupuncture therapy as a form of bioenergetic feedback, which the following case will demonstrate.

A middle-aged man came to me for a series of acupuncture treatments to learn how acupuncture worked, and to help with an almost constant low-grade flu that sapped him of much energy. The initial evaluation revealed a primary weakness in the Greater Yin energetic function (Lung and Spleen), especially the Lungs. Treatment focused on strengthening the Lung function, and the client received two further prophylactic treatments for this condition, in the fall, to help prevent an aggravation of the condition in the spring, which had been occurring for some years.

When the client returned a few months later, he mentioned as an aside that he realized, after each of the previous acupuncture sessions, that his "motor wasn't running" all the time. He explained that this *motor*, of which he had been previously unaware, entailed a kind of full feeling in the abdomen and a need to constantly nibble on snacks. When asked to show where this motor was located, he pointed without hesitation to the upper left region over the spleen and pancreas. When I showed him that the initial evaluation had shown a weakness in the Greater Yin system, and pointed out that the lower branch of this system is the Spleen-energetic function, connected with the Lung-energetic function, which we had focused on in the previous series of treatments, he was greatly surprised that he had a knowledge of this imbalance, an awareness that seemed to arise directly out of the acupuncture treatment. Treatment this time focused on the Spleen-energetic weakness, with secondary tonification of the associated Lung function. When the client returned in the spring for a follow-up visit, he reported that the "motor" had stopped running, that he did not have a need to nibble all the time, and that his energy was higher.

This type of recognition, this bodily felt awareness of energetic and functional disturbances, occurs almost as a side effect of acupuncture. It is as if the stimulation of a pattern of points by the acupuncture needles prodded the bodymind not only to recollect the dysfunctional pattern but also to remember how to generate an energetic "repatterning" in order to resume more normal functioning in the zone in question. This is often sufficient to resolve many functional and psychosomatic reaction patterns; but in my experience, far greater and longer-lasting results occur if the acupuncture therapist makes intentional use of his or her own awareness of the client's energetic reaction pattern to educate the client about this pattern. If this is done properly, the client will quickly begin to recall bodily experiences and psychological symptoms and imbalances that are a part of the current pattern. The therapist's task is to integrate these recollections of being with a will to be well.

The awareness of bodymind dysfunction that develops through acupuncture therapy thus conceived leads to a recognition of underlying psychic and somatic reaction patterns and hence to alleviation or resolution of many psychosomatic, functional, and stress disturbances.

On a more fundamental level, a person may begin early to recognize his or her own psychosomatic reaction patterns and thus be in a position to alter them. Coming to view the psychosomatic complaint as a microcosm of individual ways of being and reacting in the world enables the person to learn important lessons about his or her behavior and about changing it. In some cases, such a recognition will lead the patient into a long-term therapy of psyche or soma or both, resulting in changes on levels more profound than that of the original bodymind complaint. However, it is not wise to force a patient with a psychosomatic or functional complaint into long-term therapy, as this often results in a dependency that proves negative to both the patient and the therapist.

The psychosomatic complaint offers the bodymind-energetic therapist privileged access to a core aspect of the person as a whole. Neglecting the presenting complaint in favor of a broad view of the whole person may result in the patient's losing the opportunity to learn something important about his or her bodymind reactions without becoming dependent on the therapy or the therapist. The therapy ought not to become an end in itself. In the complex field of health maintenance and prevention, there is no room for egotistic therapists claiming the exclusive merits of their therapies but rather a need for creative collaboration among therapists of different sorts, orchestrated, as much as possible, by a responsible client.

The Stress Response

The stress response brings into play major activation of the sympathetic and parasympathetic nervous symptoms, as Alexander had already demonstrated, preparing the individual "for either fight or flight from which no physical escape takes place."[60] The common sympathetic system response to stress is a shifting of blood away from the periphery of the body (hands, feet, skin) and away from the gastrointestinal tract, under the influence of the parasympathetic system, towards the torso and head, leading to such symptoms as clammy hands; cold feet; chills up and down the spine; a knot in the stomach; dilated pupils; tightness in the throat, neck, and upper back; raised tight shoulders; shallow breathing; accelerated heart and pulse rate; a locked, rigid, or numb pelvis; contracted flexor muscles in the legs; and inhibited extensors.[61]

An almost identical reaction pattern is referred to in acupuncture-energetic terminology as constrained Liver energy with rising Yang of the Liver (the sympathetic part of the Five Element physiological function seen previously), often with a deficient Yin root and a relative excess of the Yang root of the Kidneys (the adrenals), leading to a stepped-up metabolism always ready for fight or flight. If the organism successfully meets the threat or escapes from it, a parasympathetic relaxation response will occur, with dilation of the body's smooth muscles. While the sympathetic system leads to a general excitation effect, the parasympathetic system reacts primarily on the gastrointestinal tract and breathing. When "the parasympathetic nervous system is activated in response to stress, it works in close coordination with the endocrine system," thereby affecting the endocrine glands which, like the autonomic nervous system, intimately affect psychological and somatic function.[62]

It is beyond the scope of this discussion to study the complex feedback loop of the endocrine system, but it is important to note that sympathetic activation reacts on the hormonal system and that, as has been proven, people can learn to control autonomic functions and therefore affect hormonal function itself. In regulating these functions, hormonal disorders also are affected.[63]

Dr. Hans Selye, an endocrinologist from Montreal, developed a key concept in the study of stress in 1956, which he termed the *general adaptation syndrome* (G.A.S.)[64] Simply speaking, the G.A.S. reaction to a stressor passes through three phases: *alarm, resistance,* and *exhaustion.*

During the *alarm phase,* the bodymind's entire stress reaction is called into play, with a generalized effect on psychological and physiological functioning. Adrenocortical secretion rises sharply, raising the blood pressure and producing symptoms of sympathetic system hyperactivity. One of the main tasks of the G.A.S., Pelletier notes, "is to delegate responsibility for dealing with a stressor to the organ or system most capable of handling it, seeking out and calling into action the most appropriate channel of defense."[65] There is a relationship between this reaction and the channels of defense of acupuncture energetics, and the acupuncture-energetic approach has much to teach us about the "appropriate channels of defense" involved in psychosomatic dysfunction.

The *resistance phase* leads to a decrease in adrenocortical secretion, as the particular organ-functional system best suited to dealing with the stress comes into play. Resistance to the specific stressor is very high at this point, but the rush of energy to the reaction site leaves other areas depleted, thus leading to a general decrease in overall resistance.

During *the exhaustion phase,* the organ-functional system wears out or breaks down. The adrenocortical secretions rise again as the task is shifted away from the exhausted functional system to the general system that reacts to the stress.

This process does not necessarily lead to a psychosomatic disorder. For "such artificially induced stressors as bloodletting and electric and chemical shocks, and natural ones such as high fever, may actually excite the body out of an ineffectual response, promote a transference of responsibility for defense to other areas, and stimulate the production of fresh cells to assist in this defense."[66]

Acupuncture can be seen as precisely such an "artificially induced stressor," of a minor sort, that leads to activation of the General Adaptation Syndrome on a miniature level, and almost always ends with a profound relaxation response while promoting the establishment of more effective psychosomatic energetic reactions by calling into play hitherto blocked energetic zones and pathways (the organ functions and meridians).

Since prolonged or unabated stress can lead to breakdown in a target organ or system, resulting in what Selye terms "diseases of adaptation,"[67] it is crucial to help clients to recognize their own patterns of reactivity to stress and to do something about them.

Acupuncture energetics supplies the missing link in understanding why and how a particular type of disorder tends to affect a person in a specific way, calling into play certain regions of the body as well as specific organ-energetic functions. Whereas Western behavioral psychologists are just beginning to categorize the various reaction patterns associated with stress syndromes, the acupuncture patterns have been observed and treated for more than two thousand years. Therefore, they provide very powerful images or metaphors of stress responses that can aid the modern investigator and clinician in developing a bodymind therapy that begins, not with some elaborate theory with which to explain the patient's responses, but rather with the patient and his or her own awareness of these imbalances. Such an approach leads quite quickly to the patient assuming responsibility for doing something about these dysfunctions rather than depending on the expert for help.

CHAPTER SUMMARY

Bodymind Energetics Reviewed

It has been the aim of this chapter to acquaint the reader with the major Western attempts to deal with the bodymind problem, from classic psychosomatics and phenomenological psychology to modern behavioral research.

As pointed out in Chapter 2, there are two basic ways in which one may reinforce the psychological side of acupuncture energetics for use in the West. One may retrieve and expand upon the psychological and spiritual dimensions inherent in the ancient Taoist teachings of acupuncture and Oriental medicine, as did J. R. Worsley in England. One may also add Western understandings of constitutional and psychological types to the brief psychological sketches of the ancient acupuncture texts, which Yves Requena has accomplished. Finally, one may juxtapose acupuncture-energetic theory and therapy with other concepts and practices that speak of the psychological side of bodymind reaction patterns. This has been my own direction in the current work.

The issues raised by modern Western thinkers, beginning with Freud and Nietzsche, in their attempts to approach the psychosomatic question have not been retained by orthodox medicine or psychiatry. Nor have they been confronted by the human potential movement or the holistic and alternative health movements of the past decade with the same philosophical rigor as in Europe.

As a new paradigm of health and health maintenance emerges, then, in the latter part of the twentieth century, it is of utmost importance that physicians and therapists of all types grapple with the complex relations between the psyche and the body process, so as to transform radically the ways in which people come to view their bodies, their selves, their illnesses, and their health. A real revolution in health care can come about only if the general public is brought into the center of the process. In this sense, therapists and physicians must be willing to teach as well as treat their clients, and be able to learn from them as well.

In what we have termed the bodymind-energetic approach, a comparison has been drawn between the insights and understandings of acupuncture and psychosomatics in order to arrive at a phenomenological approach to bodymind-energetic work that requires of therapist and client alike a philosophical, existential inquiry into health and disease, mind and body, and the relationship between therapist and client.

The major weakness of the Western psychological efforts to understand and treat the body/mind split is that they all privilege the mind (intellect, consciousness) over the body, and engage the client in intense mental work and consciousness-raising without a corresponding focus on the body and its complex dynamics.

A psychotherapist inspired by the classic psychosomatic approach will focus on helping the client gain insight into, and understanding of, the hidden meaning and symbolism behind the bodymind dysfunction. While this is important, most psychosomatic complexes are not resolved through understanding alone, and attention must be given to the somatic compliance corresponding to the psychological conflict involved in each case.

Likewise, a phenomenological psychologist may help a person describe, in his or her own terms, the nature of the bodymind imbalances and problems, but nothing in the approach necessarily recognizes the need to do more than talk. The necessity of reaching a bodymind integration *in the body* of the client is rarely ever addressed.

Finally, while behavioral therapists focusing on the stress response have directed their attention to the body and the physiological underpinnings of bodymind complaints, they have erred in the opposite direction by almost totally ignoring the need for an understanding of the meaning of illness and the role of the psyche.

In the first case, understanding is privileged as the sole source for healing, whereas in the second case, physiological alterations are believed to be sufficient. In neither is there a concerted effort to achieve bodymind integration. Therefore, the body/mind split of Western civilization continues to influence the way in which we learn about, and treat, our bodies and ourselves.

The benefit of introducing an Eastern perspective, that of acupuncture energetics, which does not stem from a duality between body and mind, is manifold.

Acupuncture energetics provides us with a detailed geographic atlas of somatic energetic zones with which to situate our clients' complaints. In this way, symptoms and ailments that previously have been diagnosed and treated as many different complaints are shown to possess a primary unity and to adhere to a specific energetic disharmony. When combined with a bodymind-integrative perspective, acupuncture assumes the proportions of a modern behavioral therapy capable of awakening a deep recognition, on the part of the patient, of body/mind splits and somatic energetic patterns of dysfunction, even before specific complaints have developed. The benefit of a preventive therapy that also enables the patient to assume more responsibility for his or her own healing is inherent in such a practice of acupuncture therapy.

The images and metaphors of acupuncture energetics—Water unable to control Fire in a case of hypertension with insomnia, Rising Liver Fire due to a deficiency in the Yin Root of the Kidney in a case of hyperthyroidism, Liver invading the Spleen in a case of a stomach ulcer, deficient Energy of the Kidneys and Lung-energetic functions in a case of asthma—stir the patient's own images of body/mind disharmony. Intervention at the level of such body/mind imbalances, with a judicious placement of needles, prods the bodymind to a higher level of functioning, resulting in an energetic repatterning that is capable of bringing great transformations.

Energetic changes occur at a level that underlies somatic or psychic functioning, and hence open the way for bodymind integration.[68]

Ultimately, acupunture brings the question of energy back into Western medicine and Western psychology, where it has been missing for a long time. The bodymind-energetic approach, with its combined use of Western psychosomatic imagery and understanding and acupuncture energetics, represents my own way, as an acupuncture therapist grounded in Western philosophy and psychology, to aim for bodymind integration in those with whom I work.

In the second half of this book I shall discuss the various systems of the bodymind from a phenomenological, bodymind-energetic perspective, beginning with the surface, the skin, moving on to the various major organ-functional units, and finishing with the musculoskeletal support system. It is hoped that this phenomenological perspective of bodymind functioning will move students, practitioners, and patients of the various forms of medicine and therapy to forge their own images of bodymind integration.

In the next chapter, we shall return to Groddeck's notion of the "will to be well." Any bodymind approach belonging to the new paradigm of health must begin with the bodymind's amazing capacity for self-healing. This shifts the locus of power in the healing relationship from the doctor or therapist to the patient, who becomes his or her own doctor. The bodymind-energetic approach attempts to restore the internal healer, for "[w]e are doctors almost before we are beings. Our cells know; they stand as magical sages and midwives at our birth, doing the impossible from matter."[69]

NOTES

1. F. Alexander, *Psychosomatic Medicine*, p. 54.
2. For further discussion of this subject, see Julian Kenyon, *21st Century Medicine*. Wellingborough, Northamptonshire; Rochester, Vermont, Thorsons Publishing Group, 1986, chapter 3.
3. Capra, *The Turning Point*, p. 317.
4. Ibid, p. 317.
5. Ibid, p. 318.
6. Ibid, p. 318.
7. Ibid, p. 318.
8. Ibid, p. 318.
9. Ibid, p. 318.
10. Weil, *Health & Healing*, p. 57.
11. Franz Alexander, *Psychosomatic Medicine*, p. 50.
12. Günter Ammon, *Psychoanalysis and Psychosomatics*. New York, Springer Publishing Co., 1979.
13. As quoted in Ammon, p. 6.
14. Ibid, pp. 15–16.
15. Ibid, p. 18.
16. Ibid, p. 19.
17. Ibid, p. 20.
18. Cf. Ammon, p. 261.
19. As quoted in Ammon, pp. 27–28.
20. See Ammon, pp. 29–32.
21. Ibid., p. 29.
22. Cf. Ammon, pp. 29–30.
23. Cf. Chapter 2.
24. See Ammon, p. 35.
25. Franz Alexander, *Psychosomatic Medicine*, pp. 41–43.
26. Ibid., p. 42.
27. Ibid., p. 51.
28. Ibid.
29. Ibid, pp. 51–52.
30. Ibid, p. 52.
31. Ibid.
32. Ibid, p. 59.
33. Ibid., pp. 59–60.
34. Ibid, pp. 60–61.
35. Ibid, p. 67.
36. Ibid, as quoted by Ammon, p. 56.
37. Ibid, p. 57.
38. As quoted in Ammon, p. 59, emphasis ours.

39. Gilles Deleuze and Feliz Guattari, *Anti-Oedipus: Capitalism and Schizophrenia,* translated from the French by Robert Hurley, Mark Seem, and Helen R. Lane. New York, Viking Press, 1983, cf. Chapters 1 and 2.
40. *Psychoanalysis and Psychosomatics,* p. 62.
41. Ibid, p. 63.
42. Ammon, p. 70.
43. Ibid, p. 72.
44. *Anti-Oedipus,* pp. 7–8.
45. Ammon, p. 77.
46. Ibid, p. 77.
47. Ibid, p. 81.
48. Ibid, p. 82.
49. It is beyond the scope of this brief summary to explore the often subtle differences between phenomenological psychiatry and existential analysis. The reader is referred to *Existence,* edited by Rollo May, Ernst Angel, Henri Ellenberger, New York, Touchstone, Basic Books, 1958, introductory chapters.
50. Ibid, pp. 32–33, quoting a statement made in 1908 before the Viennese Psychoanalytic Society dedicated, that evening, to a discussion of Nietzsche's *Genealogy of Morals.*
51. As quoted in *Existence,* p. 30.
52. Ibid, p. 52.
53. Cf. Gerald Epstein, M.D., *Waking Dream Therapy.* New York, Human Sciences Press, 1981, pp. 53–55.
54. In *Existence,* cf. pp. 97–117 for Ellenberger's detailed account of these methods.
55. Ibid, p. 116. Emphasis ours.
56. Kenneth Pelletier, *Mind as Healer, Mind as Slayer.* New York, Delta Books, 1957, pp. 3–4.
57. Ibid, p. 5.
58. Ibid, p. 7.
59. Ibid, p. 18.
60. Ibid, p. 45.
61. Ibid, p. 55.
62. Ibid.
63. For a detailed discussion of the relation between stress and the physiology of the neuroendocrine system, see Mary F. Asterita, *The Physiology of Stress.* New York, Human Sciences Press, 1985.
64. Hans Selye, *The Stress of Life.* New York, McGraw-Hill, 1956.
65. Pelletier, p. 75.
66. Ibid, pp. 95–96.
67. Ibid, p. 76.
68. Coming from an entirely different perspective, Yasuo Yuasa arrives at a similar view of meridian energetics as a "depth-psychological body." See *The Body: Toward an Eastern Mind-Body Theory.* Albany, New York, State University of New York Press, 1987, especially chapter 10, pp. 219–222.
69. Richard Grossinger, *Planet Medicine: From Stone Age Shamanism to Post-Industrial Healing.* Berkeley, California, North Atlantic Books, 1985, p. 36.

II

BODYMIND
PHENOMENOLOGY

5

Breakdown, Resistance, and the Will to Get Well

It is at work everywhere, functioning smoothly at times, at other times in fits and starts . . .[1]

Deleuze and Guattari

Bodymind energetics is neither a new form of therapy nor a new theory of therapeutics, but rather an approach to treatment involving the integrated use of acupuncture energetics and psychosomatic principles and observations. From this perspective, the bodymind is a dynamic, open, or living system that functions through constant interaction with the outside world. This interaction involves the energetic transformation of matter, characterized by continual fluctuation, reshuffling, breakdown, and regeneration. What is remarkable about a living system is its capacity for self-renewal and repair. In this light, breakdown is best understood not as disease or decay, but rather as transformation and change with the potential for regeneration. With its ability to describe energetically rather than mechanistically how living systems break down and repair themselves, the bodymind-energetic approach will further the development of a new paradigm of health maintenance based on the human capacity to regenerate and reorganize at higher levels.[2]

The modern development of this energetic perspective can be traced back to the Nietzsche-inspired concept of the "It" developed by Georg Groddeck, a prominent psychosomatic physician, at the turn of the century. In his view, the mind/body duality is a linguistic trap that prevents us from seeing the mind and body as one unit animated or driven by a life force that he termed the "It" (Das Es). While this word is identical in the original German to Freud's term for the unconscious usually translated as the "Id," Groddeck's perspective is broader. For Groddeck, "It and unconscious are two totally different concepts—the unconscious is a part of the psyche, the psyche a part of the It . . . . The It is man himself in all his vital manifestations."[3]

The It, like the Chinese concept of Qi, is the force that moves us, inhabits us, drives us. While speculation on the actual nature of the It or Qi might prove fruitless, our task in bodymind energetics is identical to Groddeck's: to understand how It moves in the bodymind and to determine the signification of this movement in the particular context and according to the specific configuration of its occurrence.

Before turning to an examination of different energetic systems of the bodymind and how they break down, a word is in order concerning the focus of the bodymind-energetic approach.

Groddeck examined many of the relevant issues in the context of his own work, which combined body therapy with an analysis of psychic dynamics.

RESISTING HEALTH

Groddeck was a medical physical therapist who never referred to himself as a psychoanalyst despite Freud's insistence that he do so. Although he had neither been analyzed nor officially studied psychoanalysis, Freud considered him to be a psychoanalyst because, as he wrote, "The discovery that transference and resistance are the most important aspects of treatment turns a person irretrievably into a member of the wild army. No matter if he calls the unconscious 'It'."[4]

Groddeck agreed with Freud that the aim of any therapy—and this is especially relevant concerning our notion of bodymind energetics—is to trace and dissolve resistances. This implies understanding the meaning of the resistances against regaining health, inherent in many illnesses, the main resistance being the will to remain ill. In this light, the therapist's task becomes one of supporting the client's will to recover by helping the client learn anew what it is like to be well.

In a personal communication Dr. Lourdes Alvarez-Klein, a physician, acupuncturist, and homeopath who first introduced me to the work of Groddeck, described the work of supporting the will to get better as follows: "The It seems to signal the consciousness through symptoms. Consciousness tries to deny, ignore, avoid or mask these manifestations for two reasons: one is that they hurt [pain, discomfort, etc.]; the other is that they represent a threat to the fixed idea of who and how we are, and confront us with the void of being something different. Pittman McGhee [a Jungian analyst] describes this as a fear of seeing what is coming in the bucket from the well of the unconscious. It is fear of disintegrating and it might be helpful to support the person during the process of realizing that disintegration is always already taking place as the bodymind tends toward a new configuration and that pain intensifies as we try to remain in the same patterns when the time and place demand different ones."

As Groddeck affirmed, "in the majority of cases by far, in my experience in more than three quarters of all cases one comes across in one's whole medical practice, it is quite sufficient to give direct support to the will to get better."[5] In breaking down resistances, the therapist must begin with the person's symptoms, the present manifestations of distress, for it would be as useless to look for the cause of disease as to try to understand the meaning of the life force (the It). This implies working with the patterns of bodymind disharmony as they present themselves phenomenologically, without any preconceived notion of a causative factor. This explains Groddeck's use of the term "It": "since it is impossible to get human thought habits away from their beaten tracks, I thought up the term It. I liked the indefiniteness about it—X would have been too mathematical, and X, moreover, demands a solution; my It, however, suggests that only a fool would try to understand it. There is nothing there to understand."[6]

In observing the patient, the bodymind therapist looks not only to overt signs and symptoms "but to everything expressed by the patient's It and perceived by the doctor's It, from the shape of the chin to the deepest emotions, from the present situation to the remote past. But we always treat a picture, a living picture and never a cause."[7]

The traditional Chinese physician is trained to perceive "patterns of disharmony"[8] in a web of signs and symptoms—patterns with no single cause, but rather a multiplicity of confluent factors producing a complex series of energetic effects. In the bodymind-energetic approach, observation of psychic configurations and the dynamic interplay between the psyche and the body process is routine, moving the latter approach away from a focus on preconceived patterns of disharmony, with an emphasis on bodymind integration.

From the bodymind-energetic perspective, the therapist's main role is to assist and guide the individual in strengthening the will to get better, on both a somatic and a psychological level. This means, additionally, that the therapist resists making himself or herself, or the therapeutics, indispensable to clients, so as not to foster dependency, and also refrains from using his or her art and knowledge to dazzle clients with labels describing their state of being or illness. For it is not possible, Groddeck reminds us, to know exactly what is wrong or even who the client really is, for "the human being in front of [us] is an arbitrary figment of (our) imagination . . . he is certainly not what (we) believe (we) can see in him."[9] The goal of our therapeutic work is not to try to know the unknowable. We will never totally know our clients, but we can empathize, and be willing to use our knowledge and our skills to help them grow stronger and take responsibility for their own development. We must be mindful of the fact that the individual who comes to us is not an isolated object for our scrutiny, but a being out of tune with the environment. Groddeck reminds us that we must not "isolate man and deny that he is animal and flower, stone and wood," for if we do we will be like a therapist or physician "who does nothing else during his whole life but look through a microscope," thus going so far as to deny "heaven, earth, the stars, since he cannot look at them through a microscope."[10]

The purpose of the bodymind-energetic approach is to multiply the perspectives from which we encounter those who seek our help, opening our senses to the person in his or her entirety, "in as many of the breadths, depths, flat and narrow bits of his nature as possible, in all the elements which all human beings share and those which seem peculiar to individuals alone . . . his shape and the shape of his limbs, his external and internal parts, and all of his functions from breathing, sleeping, moving, digesting, heart beat, to speaking, thinking, feeling."[11]

The ability to "treat the resistance is not teachable, it has to be learned, and can only be learned by treating patients; . . . the doctor's task is to liberate the patient's will to get well from all obstructions, traps, and snares."[12] One can learn with practice to recognize psychic snares and verbal traps, to free up physical and emotional blocks and obstructions—the aims of any bodymind-energetic work. Learning how to dissolve resistances is dependent on the personality and proclivities of the particular therapist and requires self-analysis and work. The effort is well worth it, for when a therapist succeeds in liberating the client's will to get well, whether through acupuncture treatment to unblock the energetic flow through a particular area of the body, through psychological understanding to help a client better comprehend the dynamics of the psyche, or through other physical or mental means, then, as Groddeck states, "recovery will come about automatically."[13]

In the discussion that follows we shall explore the major functional systems of the bodymind in order to provide therapists of psyche and soma with a bodymind-energetic phenomenology. We shall shift from the model and language of psychosomatics to that of acupuncture energetics, concluding with a bodymind-energetic evaluation of representative disorders. The combined use of these two models and languages is unavoidable from the point of view of bodymind energetics, for at this time it is still very difficult to speak the language of bodymind directly.

"Like physicists [the new practitioner] may have to be content with a network of interlocking models, using different languages to describe different aspects and levels of reality. As we use different maps when we travel to different parts of the world, we would use different conceptual models on our journeys beyond space and time, through the inner world of the psyche."[14]

And what better place to begin our investigation of the "inner world of the psyche" than by focusing on its most outward, most superficial manifestations, on the surface of the body?

NOTES

1. Gilles Deleuze and Felix Guattari, *Anti-Oedipus: Capitalism and Schizophrenia*, translated from the French by Robert Hurley, Mark D. Seem, and Helen Lane. New York, Viking Press, 1977, p. 1.
2. For an in-depth discussion of the systems view of life, see Fritjof Capra, *The Turning Point: Science, Society and the Rising Culture*, Chapter 9. New York, Bantam Books, 1982.
3. Georg Groddeck, *The Meaning of Illness*. New York, International Universities Press, 1977, pp. 15–16.
4. Ibid., p. 5.
5. Ibid., pp. 216–217.
6. Ibid., p. 11.
7. Ibid., p. 233.
8. Cf. Ted J. Kaptchuk, *The Web That Has No Weaver*, for his discussion of these patterns.
9. *The Meaning of Illness*, p. 243.
10. Ibid., pp. 243–244.
11. Ibid., p. 244.
12. Ibid., p. 226.
13. Ibid.
14. *The Turning Point*, p. 369.

6

Phenomenology of the Surface

The meaning of a rash is repulsion—and attraction.[1]

G. Groddeck

"The skin," states Franz Alexander, "constituting the surface of the body, is the somatic locus of exhibitionism."[2] Skin reactions such as blushing with embarrassment, paling with fear, and flushing with excitement betray the psychosomatic reactivity of the body surface. The most common psychosomatic skin disorders are neurodermatitis, eczema, angioneurotic edema, hives, itching, dandruff, and psoriasis, with rarer disorders ranging from skin phobias and self-induced lesions to stigmata of the crucifixion.

We in the West may associate the skin with outside, surface, touch, smooth or rough, color, rashes, acne, pimples, freckles, scars, make-up, wrinkles, dryness or oiliness, pallor, or flushing. With a little more effort, we may think of associations such as stroking and caressing, tickling and hurting, itching and clawing. We may even think of the skin of the mother, the mouth–breast connection. And yet it is much more than that. The skin, the surface of the body, is, as Flanders Dunbar noted, "a means of intercommunication between the inner and outer worlds . . . the boundary of the body as related to the environment."[3] The skin is a container, an envelope that binds the bodymind, the web of matter that holds one together. This is epitomized by the child who believes that if the belly-button were to burst, his or her being would escape.

While our inner being, spirit, or soul is contained and protected by

152

the outer skin layer, our outer being or Ego is, as Freud states in *The Ego and the Id*, first of all a body-ego, or the projection of an image on the surface. The complex relationship between the infant's skin and the skin of the mother, and the dynamic unfolding of the infant's sense of what is inside and what is outside, bespeaks a phenomenology of separation and oneness that is at the core of the bodymind process. With the severing of the umbilical cord, the infant's flesh is forever separate from that of the mother. It is no wonder that the dream of a perfect reunion is intermingled with the fantasy of blissful loss of Self in the arms of a lover, where boundaries blur and one's Self is lost within an Other. Here the distinctions between Self and Other, between life and death, between being bound and being boundless, are lost. As paradoxical as it may seem, a key aspect of our being, then, is not to be found in some deep recess of the body, but rather on the surface, where the social "Me" takes hold and gains coherence.

SURFACE PROJECTIONS

The initial emergence of the ego or social Self, as a body-ego or body-image projected onto the surface of the body, was a ground-breaking concept developed by Freud in *The Ego and the Id*.[4] In this important work, Freud postulated the relationships between the unconscious, the preconscious, and the conscious, and between the Id, the Superego, and the Ego. Freud's mechanistic concept of the psyche and mental energy is tamer than Groddeck's concept of the It, thus allowing it to exist within the confines of "science." While Groddeck postulated that the social Me (the ego) was inhabited and driven by forces that were unknown and to a large extent uncontrollable (the It), Freud's Id was the aspect of mind or spirit that only behaves as if it were not conscious.[5] Thus, the unruly Id can be tamed by a vigilant Ego, which, being inferior in strength, must actually borrow force from the Id and then use it to control the Id.[6]

The Ego, then, learns to transform the Id's will into action, appropriating this will and this action as its own. The Ego is "that part of the Id which has been modified by the direct influence of the external world,"[7] and the Ego makes use of its communication with the external world to control the forces of the Id and satisfy the desires of the Id in socially acceptable ways (Reality Principle). The Id, on the other hand, unconcerned with the rules that constitute external reality, strives only to fulfill its own desires (Pleasure Principle). The importance of the body itself, and especially its surface, is crucial to an understanding of the relationship between Ego and Id, for the body can give rise not only to external perceptions but also to internal ones.

The body as a surface "is seen like any other object, but to the *touch* it yields two kinds of sensations, one of which may be equivalent to an internal perception."[8] In the psychophysiology of Freud's day, the importance of the body as a privileged object of direct perception was explained in part by the role of localized discomfort in painful illness, where the perception of organ pain added to the knowledge of the body.[9] Thus, the initial development of a sense of self derives from the bodymind's experience in infancy of the body and its functions, beginning with the perceived surface, floating as it were in a sea of other objects—the mother's face, the father's moustache, the painted bird on the wall, the infant's own hand, the mother's breast, the infant's feet. On the undifferentiated surface of the infant's body, objects alight but do not always succeed in taking hold, for the surface is ruled by the forces of the Id. "The ego is first and foremost a bodily ego; it is not merely a surface entity, but is itself the projection of a surface."[10]

The surface of the body, thus defined by Freud, accurately depicts the normal, well-behaved Ego. This surface, as he demonstrates brilliantly in his analysis and treatment of neuroses, is a surface on which vivid representations of all sorts are projected. Faced with distorted body images or with bodily symptoms, the psychoanalyst tries to help the patient arrive at an interpretation of these bodily signs. This bringing to consciousness of the meaning of body signs and symptoms is crucial in the psychoanalytic treatment of psychosomatic disorders. The surface as depicted by Freud, where the social self (the Ego) finds its meaning, is a relatively calm surface, where the force of the Id may break through occasionally, producing a rash on an elbow, a tic near an eye, or even, in a severe case, the stigmata of the crucifixion. Unlike Groddeck, and Nietzsche before him, who viewed the forces of the It as forces that inhabit and drive the body and the Ego, Freud arrived at a calmer notion, that of an Ego which merely represents, on its own surface, these forces. This conception of the surface holds true for neurosis, perhaps, but not for psychosis. In schizophrenia, for example, the It is constantly at work, making its force felt. There is nothing calm about Groddeck's surface, where a painful knee that is red and inflamed not only *represents* a conflict to be interpreted, but also *is* an experience in the body that must be felt and lived through. The surface of the psychotic, where armies and lightning and wild animals prey, is not a mere *reflection of images* and representations, but also, and more dynamically, *a field of forces* and a play of energy. Taking the schizophrenic process (and not the hospitalized schizophrenic) as a starting point, Gilles Deleuze and Felix Guattari postulate a notion of forces and flows in the bodymind akin to Groddeck's. They suggest that in the neurotic and even in the average person, the body is a surface teeming with flows of desire, passion, anger, and fear, all of which are productive.[11] Freud's understanding of the body was influenced by a mechanistic bio-chemical model, rather than an energetic model. Hence his body was organized in a meaningful way, with every part assigned a function and a meaning. If we look at the body as a force field, there is no mind/body split, just as there is no split between humanity and Nature, such that all the forces of nature and the cosmos invade and drive us, just as in Groddeck's view, for our body is a reflection of the forces that inhabit and drive it. The surface of the body is seen in this view not as a projected image of the mother's body, but as a productive field, where events occur as a constellation of elements arranged in a series. In the face of such productions, the issue is not only, or not even, what this particular body-as-event *means*, but what it *does*—what *effect* it has, how it *behaves*, *moves*, and *works*. This view of the body portrays the surface as contiguous with the whole of society and the environment. Such a phenomenological view of the surface as force field frees us of the mechanistic model that confined Freud: "A schizophrenic out for a walk is a better model than a neurotic lying on the analyst's couch. A breath of fresh air, a relationship with the outside world."[12]

Rather than a model of the surface (Ego) in opposition to the interior (Id), Deleuze and Guattari propose a model of body-as-force-field, as we saw briefly in Chapter 4, on whose surface two types of force interact; forces of attraction and forces of repulsion. Attractive forces work to pull objects into the body, to incorporate them into the body's own processes of organization and transformation (desiring-production). Repelling forces, on the other hand, are forces that resist organization, that repel objects from the surface (anti-production, or the "body without organs"): "The body without organs is not the proof of an original nothingness, nor is it what remains of a lost totality. Above all, it is not a projection; it has nothing to do with the body itself, or with an image of the body. *It is the body without an image.*"[13] This experience of the body without an image, which directly contradicts Freud's concept of "body-image," is simply the experience of the body as force field, as a free flow of active and reactive forces, of fluctuations and transformations, in which entropy is part of the process. This image of the bodymind and of psychic forces is consistent with the new energetic paradigm discussed earlier. In our attempts to understand the breakdowns of the bodymind, whether as therapists working primarily through the body or therapists working through the psyche, we must not be content solely with restructuring the body or reorganizing our clients' understanding of their psychic conflicts.

The issue is not only to help our clients become more balanced, to develop a more integrated bodymind, but also to enable them to understand the nature of their disorganizations, their imbalances, their body without organs.

Freud's surface is appropriately calmed, for it is dominated by the forces of reason. Working from within a mind/body duality, Freud thought that the task of the psychoanalyst was to assist in controlling the body (Id) by exertion of the mind (Ego) through the intellectual work of interpreting and understanding the meaning of the Id's images and projections on the surface of the body. The energetic view (Groddeck, Deleuze, Guattari) of the surface is more turbulent and depicts a body forced to adapt to the pressures of the social world and the environment—to become bound at the surface by societal and familial rules, taboos and restrictions, to respond constantly to environmental factors and external stressors. It is not enough to understand the meaning of body symptoms or defenses; we must also work to help our clients experience what these defenses do, how they work, and what purpose they fill in the economy of the bodymind's energetic productions. Wilhelm Reich realized this when he turned toward an analysis of what he termed "character armor." He recognized that psychological interpretation was insufficient and that in order to free up the surface of the body (psychosomatic disturbances) one also had to touch this body, to make it aware of its presence, to make the bodymind feel its constrictions and manifest a will to break through these restrictions to achieve freedom.

The aim of a bodymind-energetic approach is to focus not only on psychic defenses, but also on surface, body defenses, realizing that the two always occur simultaneously.

MARKS ON THE BODY

Classic psychosomatic literature on the skin emphasizes that scratching is a hostile drive, which because of guilt feelings is deflected from its original target and directed against the Self. Alexander cites the case, which we shall refer back to in our own case at the end of this chapter, of a woman with severe bouts of neurodermatitis. The lesions occurred on the face and the upper and lower extremities and were eczematous, with discrete, red, raw itching areas. The woman scratched violently, especially while asleep, until the lesions wept and bled, leaving her disfigured. The condition had been present off and on throughout her life. She had first developed eczema a week after her birth. Her mother had been distraught during her pregnancy by the accidental death of her son and the ensuing divorce initiated by her husband. The patient was shy and backward in school, and felt different from the rest of the children because she had no father. In college, Alexander continues, she blossomed socially and formed close attachments to men. They were always broken off with the appearance of a severe attack of this skin condition. After a short period of analysis, the woman realized that the eruptions were related to guilt feelings and depression following sexual relations with men after she learned they had no intention of marrying her. Alexander notes that she searched for father substitutes in these men, and had oral cravings and "a wish for musculocutaneous cuddling."[14] Faced with frustration of these desires, she reacted invariably with guilt and hostility, which found expression thus: "all men are bastards!" This guilt turned against the Self and led to a projection of the initial effects on the skin surface itself. The more severe the hostility, the more violently she scratched herself, often leading to actual disfigurement and initiating a vicious cycle of shame, humiliation, and rejection. Feeling unloved and unlovable at such moments, she would try to get closer to her mother (oral cravings for love-nourishment). Since this always failed, she would sink into a depression and become aggressive, precipitating a breaking of close ties with women and men friends (since she was unlovable), a shutting off of her emotions and desires, and finally a clearing up of the skin. After three years of analysis, Alexander concludes, she gained control of this psychosomatic reaction pattern. She married, and the skin condition remained clear. Alexander emphasizes that in such conditions, somatic treatment is often essential, especially at night when itching is most pronounced. While he was referring to the application of ointments or the use of medications, a judicious use of acupuncture therapy to regulate energetic circulation in the meridian zones involved might have led to more rapid improvement in the condition as well as to a clearer understanding of the reaction pattern involved. Intervention solely on the level of the psyche is not sufficient, especially in the face of recalcitrant conditions such as this case of eczema. The use of suppressant medications drives the condition away from the surface, artificially resolving and therefore delaying the true resolution of precisely those conflicts that have made their way to the surface. In situations like this, physical-energetic therapies will be of great use. The combined use of psychotherapy and energetic therapy directed at the physical body would have the aim of helping the bodymind flow more appropriately on the surface.

Over 50 years ago, Flanders Dunbar, a pioneer in psychosomatics, decried the inability or refusal of the dermatologists of her day to perceive the psychological aspect of such skin disorders, despite the fact that there was an abundant literature on the psychogenesis of specific skin conditions. A quick look at today's literature will show that awareness of the psychogenic nature of skin disorders has all but disappeared from the common medical teachings, as though the skin were simply a surface to be kept blemish-free.

In *Emotions and Bodily Changes*, Dunbar discusses the phenomenology of the skin as "a means of intercommunication between the inner and outer worlds."[15] The skin is alternatively experienced as sensitive to cold, heat, pain, itching, sexual pleasure, and burning, as ugly or beautiful, red or pale, but also, and more profoundly, "as the boundary of the body as related to the environment."[16] Almost all human experience is interconnected with a sensory, optical, and aromatic experience of the skin. Manufacturers of perfume understand this, as do beauticians. Adorning the skin with scars, tattoos, scents, or jewels is a universal custom, a means of linking a person to his or her crowd, environment, and "age."

Anthropological studies of native cultures abound in descriptions of ritualistic scarring or marking of the skin, as an initiation rite meant to introduce the adolescent into his or her cultural place in life. These cultures are always oral, but as Deleuze and Guattari show, this is not because they are illiterate. For while they may lack a written language on tablets or paper, they do not lack a graphic system: "a dance on the earth, a drawing on a wall, *a mark on the body* are a graphic system, a geo-graphism, a geography."[17] This graphic system immediately relates the person undergoing the ritual to the environment and tribe, permanently engraving the structures of kinship in the flesh itself: "In the rituals of affliction the patient does not speak, but receives the spoken word. He does not act, but is passive under the graphic action; he receives the stamp of the sign. And what is his pain if not a pleasure for the eye that regards it, the collective or divine eye that is not motivated by any idea of revenge, but is alone capable of grasping the subtle relationship between the sign engraved in the body and the voice issuing from a face—between the mark and the mask."[18]

We moderns doubtless feel far removed from this "theater of cruelty." And yet, are we so different in circumcising our boys, in painting the nails of our girls or piercing their ears, in covering our bodies with stylish clothes or lavish make-up? We also wear the mask of our social self. Our surface appearance mingles in a complex fashion with our sense of identity and belonging to a particular time, class, political and social movement, or ethnic style. When symptoms come to mar this carefully kept surface/mask, we may well suspect the work of primitive forces and the existence of primal conflicts ready to burst through the pores. The nature of these forces, the meaning of these signs, must be grasped by our clients in their own terms.

PROTECTION AGAINST EXTERNAL INVADERS

An entirely different sense of how the surface of the body acts and reacts with its environment will be gained by looking at skin disorders from an acupuncture-energetic perspective.

In the acupuncture-energetic framework, the skin is the outside fortress wall that protects the valuable internal organ-functions against external invasions of the elements—cold, wind, rain, dampness, dryness, the red-hot sun. It is where inside and outside unite, as we saw in the discussion of meridian energetics in Chapter 2, that is, where an external meridian is connected to an internal branch that traverses its corresponding organ and fuels its corresponding functions and activities.

For practitioners of acupuncture therapy, the skin is associated with the site of the circulation of defensive energy (Wei Qi), which controls the opening and closing of the pores in conjunction with the Lungs, to regulate temperature in the body by releasing heat or keeping out cold; the reflection of internal energetic functioning; the locus of colors and odors that may guide an acupuncture diagnosis; the site of the most superficial meridian system, the tendino-muscular meridians, involved in the majority of pain syndromes; the zone to palpate and treat to regulate internal energetic dysfunctions; the area ruled by the Greater Yang meridian system of Small Intestine and Bladder, which covers more surface territory than the other systems; the deeper aspect of the skin, which is called the "Form" or the "flesh" in Chinese Medicine, which is under the control of the Greater Yin meridian system of Spleen and Lung. In brief, the skin is the zone where internal defensive energy flows to ward off external invaders, a zone of intense defensive activity and energetic conflict, the stage upon which all acupuncture therapy is played. Therefore, it is not surprising that acupuncture places great importance on the skin and the surface of the body. For it is on the skin that meridian energetics are most visible and palpable, with different textures, hot or cold areas, tight or loose flesh and musculature, congested or weak regions, and sensitivity at acupuncture points all guiding data for acupuncture diagnostic investigation and treatment planning.

One of the most striking things about the acupuncture approach to the skin and its disorders is the importance given to the precise location of the disorder as indicative of the disturbed, specific, energetic systems.

In *The Web That Has No Weaver*, Ted Kaptchuk relates an incident that took place in a Chinese medical dermatology class early in his

Chinese medical studies in Macau. The professor was discussing shingles, a painful skin disorder with vesicular eruptions on the the trunk of the body or face. In Kaptchuk's words: "Dr. Yu began to describe how an eruption of the face indicated a different disease process than did an eruption on the trunk. I raised my hand and asked incredulously how two identical eruptions (identical from the Western viewpoint and hence my own) could signify different disease processes simply because of their location. My teacher, amused by my confusion, smiled and explained that an eruption appearing on the face was different from an eruption on the lower trunk because its relationship to the entire body was different."[19] In other words, if a skin disorder develops on the face, it must involve dysfunctions in the meridians that flow through that region, just as a skin disorder whose symptoms manifest on the back involve an energetic disturbance of meridians that run down the entire back and back of the legs, or as a rash along the inner aspect of the legs may indicate disturbance of the three Yin meridians of the lower extremities that energize these zones.

The first energetic system that comes to mind in acupuncture with regard to skin function is the Metal (Lung/Large Intestine) system. The Lungs have the energetic function of controlling the opening and closing of the pores and the circulation of defensive energy at the surface, and the Large Intestine function controls elimination, which, when blocked, often leads to manifestations through the pores. Actually, skin energetics are more complicated than this; they involve several levels of interaction, from the superficial circulation of defensive energy in the tendino-muscular superficial meridians to the circulation of nourishing energy and blood in the veins and arteries.

Defensive energy (Wei-Qi) is important in understanding the energetics of the skin, for it is controlled by the Lung function as well as those of Kidney Yang and the Liver, and is intimately connected with the sympathetic system and external "fight-or-flight" mechanisms. The role of the Blood (Xue) in skin energetics is also of prime importance, and includes the functions of these systems: the Heart (the "Sea of Blood"); the Liver, which stores blood; and the Spleen, which regulates Blood and maintains it in the vessels. Thus, the role of the Greater Yin (Lung and Spleen functions) becomes important, as it is the zone that opens to the exterior, to the skin, owing to the Lung-energetic functions, and to the flesh and connective tissue, owing to the Spleen-energetic functions, under the sway of an ongoing struggle and interplay between internal and external factors and forces. While the aggressing pathogenic factors (wind, cold, dampness, and so forth) attempt to bypass defensive energy in order to penetrate into the blood, the blood tries to rid itself of the intrusive pathogenic agents with the help of this defensive, protective energy, the success of the latter depending on the strength of the Greater Yin system.[20]

An external disorder will manifest at the level of the superficial capillaries, with acute, violent or intense (Yang) signs that are short-lived and reversible, most often affecting the Wood (Gallbladder or Liver) systems. These Wood skin disorders will involve a sympathetic system reaction pattern, such as allergic skin disorders like hives, pruritus, or acute outbreaks of contact eczema. An internal disorder of the skin system will attack one prone to a parasympathetic reaction pattern, manifesting in an entirely different fashion, with signs of a deep disorder of blood regulation and defensive energy. This type of disorder is Yin in nature, of an insidious onset, chronic, and more difficult to treat. It will appear most commonly in Greater Yin (Lung and Spleen) and Sunlight Yang (Stomach and Large Intestine) systems, and include such disorders of the skin as constitutional eczema, psoriasis, and collagen disorders.

A survey of skin disorders of the sympathetic type (Wood, Liver and Gallbladder) as presented by Requena shows that those involving sudden sensitivity, such as hives, contact eczematous disorders, and edema, are related to deficiency of the Liver function in producing blood, and are connected to the influence of wind and heat. As we saw earlier, wind relates to moving or sudden symptoms, hence the onset of these conditions will be rapid. The blood will be hot (hence the appearance of dry scalp and dandruff), and treatment will be aimed at cooling the blood, calming the Liver wind, and easing the spirit to quell the itching.

Chronic skin disorders will occur in those with energetic dysfunction in the Earth (Spleen and Stomach) and Metal (Lung and Large Intestine) functions, that is, in the Sunlight Yang and Greater Yin systems. When a skin disorder is related to the Large Intestine function, it will be accompanied by dark grayish skin, which will be very dry and tend to grow wrinkled early. The most chronic and most difficult skin disorders to treat in Chinese medicine are attributed to dysfunction of the Lung and Spleen system (Greater Yin).

A relationship may be posited between the energetic phases of acupuncture and the Freudian psychosexual stages as follows: the Earth relates to the oral stage (Stomach and Spleen–Pancreas functions), and the Metal phase relates to the anal stage (Large Intestine and Lung functions). Therefore the disorders of Earth will involve issues of loving and giving nourishment, being loved and receiving nourishment—that is, conflicts over dependence and independence. Disorders of Metal will involve issues of separation and individuation. The first separation, departure from the womb (Yin sphere) at birth, leads to tension related to nurturing. The second separation, involved in weaning and learning self-control of muscular movements such as grasping and holding—and, most notably, sphincter control— occurs during the sphere of Metal functioning (Large Intestine/Lung functions). It is connected, in Five Phase energetic theory, with grief and weeping. The colicky baby who develops skin rashes and intestinal complaints within the first two years of life is manifesting a common example of an Earth-Metal system disturbance that must be treated accordingly.

The skin is dependent on the functions of Greater Yin (Lung/Spleen functions), which serve to externalize internal conflicts.[21] Contrary to acute Wood disorders, those of Greater Yin will be chronic and will involve the deeper aspect of the skin functions. They include such common problems as acne, chronic eczema, psoriasis, diabetic skin disorders, and collagen skin disorders. The Chinese classics state that the Lung-energetic functions nourish the skin. According to Five Phase theory, sadness and grieving injure the Lung energetic function, and hence indirectly the skin. Skin disorders related to separation and grief, especially over the loss of a loved one, are of this nature. Such conditions are also often accompanied by asthma, attesting to the Lung-Large Intestine energetic connection. While this connection has no Western physiological explanation, it has frequently been noted in the psychoanalytic literature on psychosomatic skin and respiratory disturbances. The Chinese medical classics also state that the skin "fears" pungent flavors and heat because, according to Five Phase energetics, Fire can injure Metal, and therefore heat can injure the lungs and the skin. Psychosomatic skin disorders in an individual with a predisposition to Metal dysfunction will arise as a result of a multiplicity of factors, including grieving, dryness or heat, an inability to eliminate physically or emotionally, and an excess of pungent foods. Finally, skin disorders affecting a large area of the body, especially the back and forehead, will require treatment of the Greater Yang (Bladder and Small Intestine) system, as it regulates these zones.

It is not the purpose of this book to provide a detailed discussion of acupuncture-energetic skin pathology and treatment.[22] Suffice it to say that in speaking of the energetics of the skin, acupuncture therapy focuses not only on the nature of the disorder (dry, moist, hot, or cold) but also on its location along specific meridian pathways related to specific functional systems. Each functional system brings into play an entire series of Five Phase correspondences that includes emotional, behavioral, and environmental factors. Therefore, treatment of skin disorders in acupuncture therapeutics is aimed not only at relieving distressing symptoms such as itching, dryness, or pain, but also at regulating the core energetic imbalance. This energetic regulation often enables the individual to gain greater awareness of the deeper significance of what only appears to be a superficial disorder. At the same time, a description of the precise energetic disharmony, accompanied by palpation of the affected energetic zones, will clarify how and why the disorder affects specific areas and functions of the bodymind and not others. This sets the stage for a bodily felt recognition of the disturbed zones and potential for restoring harmony to them.

For example, a person who learns that his chronic skin condition affects the Large Intestine meridian, that the Large Intestine energetic function is to eliminate, physically and mentally, and finally that the Metal phase is strongly influenced by grieving, might well have gained an image or metaphor sufficiently powerful to link together both the meaning of his father's death when he was a child and the psychosomatic manifestations of this loss and grieving in the weeping sores of his bodymind. The strength of the acupuncture-energetic explanation is that it can pinpoint with precision the psychosomatic-energetic functional system involved, thereby permitting an individualized treatment on the physical and psychological levels. Combined with the appropriate psychological therapy or counseling, the acupuncture-energetic approach is of significant value in many forms of functional and psychosomatic skin disorders.

THE PHENOMENOLOGY OF ECZEMA

It seems appropriate to conclude this discussion of the phenomenology of skin energetics with a brief look at the case that first spurred my attempt to develop the bodymind-energetic approach.[23]

A woman in her middle 20s sought acupuncture treatment for what had been diagnosed as chronic eczema. Initially occurring only on the hands, the condition worsened over the two months immediately preceding her first acupuncture treatment, spreading all along her arms, up her chest and neck, and over her cheeks, with the beginnings of a rash along the outer aspect of her legs as well. The client also complained of alternating bouts of diarrhea and constipation, clicking in her ears, and occasional heart palpitations. A graduate student in social work, she had undergone psychotherapy and used homeopathic and vitamin therapies with mild success in treating her skin condition. At the intake interview she voiced the opinion that her skin symptoms were due to food allergies and were not emotionally related.

The acupuncture evaluation revealed primary deficiencies in the Water and Fire systems (Kidney/Bladder and Heart/Small Intestine) as well as secondary hyperactivity in the Earth and Metal phases (Stomach and Large Intestine, Sunlight Yang functions, specifically).

Initial treatment of the underlying Water/Fire disharmony brought only slight improvement, and the client returned somewhat discouraged. In the second session, treatment was directed toward the hyperactive Stomach/Large Intestine functions and led to a marked clearing of the skin that lasted five days. At the start of the third session, I was compelled to reiterate the energetic and psychological function of the Small Intestine Official, which, somatically, is to "separate pure from impure," and which, on the psychological level, has to do with sorting out what is important from what is unimportant, and of the energetic function of the Large Intestine, which is elimination, and has to do with the ability to hold on to and let go of emotional experiences appropriately.

Acupuncturists will be interested to note that her disorder pointed to a multiplicity of factors, including an inherited or constitutional deficiency in the Water Phase (Kidney-Bladder), precipitating overactivity in the Fire Phase (Heart-Small Intestine), with palpitations, inappropriate laughter, and rapid speech as well as problems with elimination anally and through the skin. A picture of this client's energetic dynamics emerged: deficiency of Water leading to a hyperactivity of Fire (due to an inability in Water to properly control Fire along the Control Cycle of the Five Phases), resulting in Metal being injured by this Fire overactivity (Fire destroys Metal along the Destruction Cycle). The main functions disturbed were the Yang functions of Small Intestine (Fire) and Large Intestine (Metal), which explained the past bouts of constipation and diarrhea.

After I explained the bodymind energetics to the client, she was instructed to reflect, while the acupuncture needles were in place, on this bodymind-energetic pattern.

As the needles were removed at the end of this third session, she voiced the realization that the foods she had been reacting to "allergically" were precisely those she had eaten during "the last supper" with her lover before he abruptly broke off their relationship. Admitting that she had experienced very little emotion in reaction to this event and concluding that perhaps her skin condition was her way of holding on to him, she finally recognized the psychological component of her condition. Before she left the office, I asked her to read the case in Alexander's *Psychosomatic Medicine* of a woman suffering a similar case of eczema (discussed in detail in the preceding pages) to see if it might be of some use to her. As she left, after reading the case, she simply said that many things had become clarified.

Essentially symptom-free after another six sessions, she was sufficiently impressed by this experience to consider the possibility of combining her future career as a psychotherapist with referrals to acupuncture for her clients, in order to treat body as well as mind.

Her excitement about a combined use of psychotherapy and acupuncture led me to reflect at great length on the deficiencies of the acupuncture approach concerning treatment of the psychological side of my clients' complaints, and I began to read widely in the psychosomatic literature, which had fascinated me in my graduate studies.

As I read I discovered parallels between the psychosomatic perspective and acupuncture observations of energetic dysfunction, and began to utilize the images of psychosomatics as educational tools in my work. These images, combined with a detailed discussion of the acupuncture-energetic patterns involved in each case, served as powerful devices in opening the context of my work with patients to include what I now term a bodymind-integrative perspective. As they learned, they asked what they could do with these images, which led me to seek training in other appropriate bodymind methods (Ericksonian hypnotherapy, reframing, neurolinguistic programming, imaging). This in turn led to a combined use of these methods, always used to reinforce the patients' own, bodily felt sense of their problems brought about by the acupuncture therapy itself.

In many instances, the failure of psychotherapy as a therapeutic method in the treatment of psychosomatic disorders can be rectified by incorporating an acupuncture-energetic perspective that tackles these problems from the somatic-energetic, as well as the psycho-energetic side.

For it is clear to any psychotherapist who makes a real attempt to treat somatic problems that physical symptoms are rarely shed by understanding alone. Such functional disturbances of the bodymind often require direct attention, not merely at the deep psychic level, but also directly at the surface where the psyche's complicated dynamics are visible in the dramatic signs they produce.

NOTES

1. *The Meaning of Illness*, p. 202.
2. Franz Alexander, *Psychosomatic Medicine*. New York, W. W. Norton, 1950, p. 164.
3. Flanders Dunbar, *Emotions and Bodily Changes*. New York, Columbia University Press, 1935, p. 373.
4. Sigmund Freud, *The Ego and the Id*, translated from the German by Joan Riviere and James Strachey. New York, W.W. Norton, 1960, pp. 14–17.
5. Ibid, p. 13.
6. Ibid, p. 15.
7. Ibid., p. 15.

8. Ibid.
9. Ibid., pp. 15–16.
10. Ibid., p. 16.
11. Gilles Deleuze, Felix Guattari, *Anti-Oedipus*, pp. 1–10.
12. Ibid, p. 2.
13. Ibid, p. 8 (emphasis ours).
14. *Psychosomatic Medicine*, p. 167.
15. Flanders Dunbar, *Emotions and Bodily Changes*. New York, Columbia University Press, 1935, p. 372.
16. Ibid., p. 373.
17. *Anti-Oedipus*. p. 188 (emphasis ours).
18. Ibid., p. 189.
19. *The Web That Has No Weaver*, p. xix.
20. Cf. Requena, *Terrains et Pathologie*, pp. 369–412 for a detailed discussion of these skin disorders and their treatment.
21. *Terrains et Pathologie*, Vol. II, p. 369.
22. For a detailed discussion of pathology in traditional Chinese medicine see Kaptchuk, *The Web That Has No Weaver*, pp. 321–335; for in-depth discussion of acupuncture energetic treatment of specific disorders, see Requena, *Terrains et Pathologie*, Volumes I, II, and III (currently in translation by Redwing Press, Boston); for a discussion of acupuncture treatment planning, see Mark Seem, *Acupuncture Energetics*, New York, Thorsons Inc., 1987.
23. Presented in slightly different form at a workshop at the Traditional Acupuncture Foundation's 1984 conference, September 19, 1984, and published on tape as "Acupuncture, Psychosomatics and the Psychoenergetics of the Skin," by Mark D. Seem, Ph.D., Dipl. Ac. (NCCA).

7

Phenomenology of the Upper Zone: Respiration and Circulation

God, when He created Man
Breathed into his nostrils the
Breath of life, and Man became
A Living Soul.[1]

G. R. Heyer

In the chapters to follow we shall adopt the acupuncture-energetic perspective of the internal organ-functional systems as three energetic zones, known as the "three burning spaces"or "triple heater."

In the acupuncture-energetic formulation, the "upper heater is a mist," entailing the organ-energetic functions of the Lung and Heart systems. The "mist" refers to vaporized water in the Lungs, which is circulated throughout the body by the action of the Heart circulatory function.[2] Crucial to this process is the Yang (heating) aspect of the Kidney function. The Kidney is the "child" of the Lung function, and the Kidney (Water) also controls the action of the Heart and Pericardium (Fire) functions. Receiving its energy from the Lung function, the Yang of the Kidneys transmutes the body's water into "mist," enabling these fluids to move up and circulate throughout the body. From a Western perspective, the function of this upper zone is to take in air and oxygenate blood, thereby insuring a pure circulation of nourishing fluids throughout the body. When the upper zone is properly nourished, a person is capable of great emotional warmth

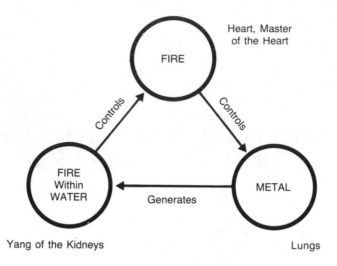

and peace of mind. If this zone is stressed, the Pericardium, also known as the "Master of the Heart" function, is called into play and works to ward off stress from the heart organ. This leads to a panic reaction pattern in which the musculature in the chest becomes hard, almost frozen, compromising the free flow of blood to the head. This muscular rigidity is like armor that the Master of the Heart places in front of the heart, leading to many non-organic cardiac symptoms. Tightness in the chest will also prevent the Lung function from performing optimally, resulting in a condition known as Fire (Heart and Master of the Heart) overcontrolling Metal (Lungs). In short, the upper zone is comprised of the energetics of Water, Fire, and Metal, which form a functional unit.

The other two zones, which we shall explore in Chapters 8 and 9, are the middle zone, comprising the Stomach, Spleen, and Liver energetic functional systems, and the lower zone, comprising the Kidney and Bladder and eliminative and reproductive energetic functions.

THE BREATH OF LIFE—RESPIRATION AND THE LUNG ENERGETIC FUNCTION

According to classic psychosomatics, the respiratory function is often affected by emotional factors. Under stress, a person's breathing becomes irregular and shallow, reducing the supply of oxygen the blood obtains in the lungs. This in turn leads to tightness in the chest and general weakness.[3] Psychosomatic texts of the 1930s often refer to the importance of diaphragmatic activity, even categorizing disorders of this function as "diaphragmatic neuroses."[4]

Breathing is the first action taken by the infant in the outside world. The sudden force placed on the lungs and diaphragm at birth (environmental stress) causes them to react by taking in "good" air and expelling "bad" air. This initial force or pressure from the outside world on the organism remains a prototype of the panic reaction to life-threatening situations in which, literally, one's breath may be taken away.

In dealing with organ function, we are rarely concerned with separate functions, but rather with all of the repercussions of this function as it interacts with associated functions. In describing the correlates of the respiratory function, Flanders Dunbar, a pioneer of psychoanalytic psychosomatics, paints a picture remarkably similar to the acupuncture-energetic view, in which the energetics of the bodymind are perceived as *fields of correlated events*. As she notes, regarding respiratory function, "it is not only the lungs that move, but mouth and nose, spinal column and shoulder girdle, the muscles of the thorax and diaphragm. All these parts participate and in their turn are influenced developmentally by respiration. There is an interaction of the respiratory apparatus, even with the abdomen and its wall and contents. What we call the bearing of the individual, psychic as well as somatic, is in closest relationship to the respiratory function."[5] It is interesting to note the correlation between this description and the acupuncture-energetic pathway of the Lung meridian itself, which commences in the solar plexus, travels to the Large Intestine, and then continues up through the diaphragm and chest to the shoulder girdle and down the arm.

The close association between cardiac and respiratory activity was observed by Paul Astruck, a psychosomatic physician, who noted that both functions "can be influenced by verbal suggestion under hypnosis. The diaphragmatic action under such influence differs from that in a waking state."[6] This, again, is in close correlation to the acupuncture-energetic view, in which air, the breath of life (*Qi*), enters the body from the cosmos, and by moving the blood (owing to the function of the upper energetic zone) gives it life.

Westerners may associate the Lung function with breathing, holding or losing one's breath, breathtaking, breathless, the rib cage, mucus, allergies, the nose and nostrils, the throat and chest, tightness in the chest, and endurance. With further prodding, we may obtain associations such as these: the first breath of life, taking in something pure and good and giving off something bad and noxious, separation from the womb, the relationship between the interior and the exterior, receiving and expelling, and so forth.

The core psychosomatic constellation of those suffering from respiratory disorders, according to Franz Alexander, is a "conflict centering around an excessive unresolved dependence on the mother."[7] This dependence upon the mother or her substitute, Alexander showed, is in marked contrast to the conflict of a person suffering gastric neurosis; the latter centers on the oral desire to be fed and loved, whereas this is more "the wish to be protected, to be encompassed by the mother or the maternal image."[8]

Gerard, a colleague of Alexander, noted that fear, anger, and anxious doubt were the most common emotions affecting respiratory function.[9]

The correlation postulated by acupuncture energetics between respiratory dysfunction and fear (where fear corresponds to the Water phase, or Kidney function) is corroborated by Alexander, who noted frequent dreams of "water symbolism" in those suffering respiratory complaints. As we shall see, the most common types of respiratory disorders in Oriental medicine are related to the energetic functions of the Liver (anger, associated with the Liver and the Wood phase, insults the Lungs and the Metal phase, in opposition to the normal control cycle;

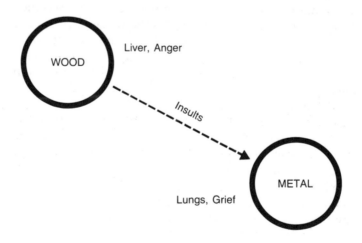

the Kidneys (fear, associated with the Kidneys and the Water phase, drains its "mother," the Lungs and the Metal phase, in opposition to the normal generation cycle);

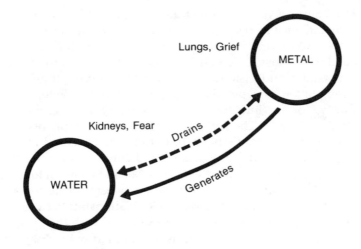

and the Spleen (anxious doubt or worry, associated with the Spleen and the Earth phase, fails to moisten and nourish, through its transporting and transforming functions, its child, the Lungs and the Metal phase; the Spleen and the Lung functions together constitute the Greater Yin unit).

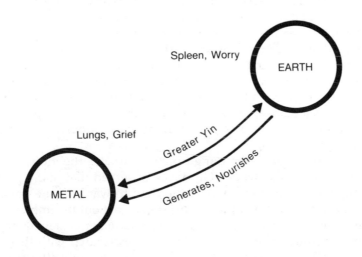

Thus, the emotions noted by Gerard and Alexander as factors in the genesis of respiratory distress are confirmed by acupuncture-energetic findings.

As several authors have demonstrated, this constellation of dependence/independence in respiratory complaints has to do with wishing to gain "protection from a person upon whom the patient depended and whose loss he feared," the fear of the loss of the mother's love "as a result of indecision and conflict between the urge to cling and the temptation to separate from her," a "lack of independence and maturity," or an "inhibition or repression of a crying that arose from anxiety or rage."[10] The generation of physical complaints in conjunction with psychic conflicts such as this was observed for thousands of years by Oriental physicians, and confirmed by the classic psychosomatic physicians whose eye for detail and focus on functional dynamics led their inquiry into the relation between psyche and soma.

Many authors have noted the dynamic relationship between confession and asthma in which confession is linked with the expiratory act of speech; surprisingly, a relationship is noted with constipation (the inability to let go linked with the inability to take in).[11] Classic psychosomatic discussions of constipation (the inability to let go) and respiratory complaints such as asthma (the fear of loss, culminating in an inability to take in) explain the *psychodynamics* linking intestinal and respiratory functions. The acupuncture-energetic viewpoint explains the *somatic energetics* involved, in which the Lung and Large Intestine functions are internally-externally related as pairs in the Metal-functional phase. Because of an inability to explain the somatic dynamics associated with psychodynamic constellations, the classic psychosomatic approach suffered in therapeutic efficacy. This was due to a bias in favor of intervention on the side of the psyche. Dunbar was alone among her colleagues in strongly advocating somatic intervention as well, and we shall show that the bodymind-energetic approach, which always intervenes on the side of the soma as well as the psyche, is a more appropriate therapy than the classic psychosomatic approach in the treatment of many psychosomatic and functional complaints.

As mentioned earlier, the Lung function situates the individual in relation to the outside world. Groddeck observed that many people use coughing, often at the start of the day, to ward off the possible evil effects of their dreams and, in this way, "cast out the impressions of their dreams and blow away the minor and major anxiety fantasies and embarrassments of the day which are associated with these."[12] This is the psychic correlate of taking in "good" air only after ridding oneself of "bad," "dirty" air. This image has proven effective in imaging techniques in which the patient imagines dark, foul air being expelled from the system to be replaced by pure bright light, thus ridding the body of mucus and restoring normal respiratory function.[13]

CONFESSION AND ASTHMA

As we have seen, the central conflict for some asthmatics is an un-resolved dependency around the person of the mother. While attempts to define a specific personality configuration for the asthmatic have proven futile, Alexander notes that "the repressed dependence on the mother is, however, a constant feature around which different types of character defenses develop."[14]

Anything, the classic psychosomatic literature maintains, that poses the threat of separation from either the protective mother or her sub-stitute, is sufficient to precipitate an attack. Sexual temptation, mar-riage, and stressful situations prompting a desire to retreat or run away are all sufficient psychic factors for the generation of asthma attacks.

Alexander does not deny the role of allergies, pointing to research showing the likelihood that in many asthmatics psychic conflicts and allergens coexist, and indicating that desensitization to either stimu-lus may suffice to end an attack. Other common factors in the genesis of asthma all revolve around a vacillation between taking in and let-ting go, such as ambivalence on the part of the mother, a combina-tion of seduction and rejection, or independence that was premature and forced on the person.[15]

Confession, Alexander notes, often helps to dissolve an asthma at-tack, as "speaking (confessing) is a more articulate use of the expira-tory act by which the adult achieves the same result as the child does by crying. He regains the love of the person upon whom he de-pends."[16]

ACUPUNCTURE ENERGETICS OF BREATH

The energetic function of the Lungs, as we saw in Chapter 2, is to direct the energetic breath of life (Qi) throughout the body by taking in air, sending it downward, and promoting the proper flow of blood from the heart. The Lung function also works to move Water down-ward to the Kidneys to circulate it around the body, especially through the pores of the skin. The Lung function controls the opening and closing of the pores, the body hair, the secretion of sweat, and the flow of protective energy to ward off external pathogenic factors. This can be expanded to include the ability to open up emotionally to the outside world, and to know when to close off and retreat. The Lung function also controls the throat, the vocal cords, and the power of the voice itself.

Energetically, the Lung function is paired with the other Metal Phase function, that of the Large Intestine, which flows internally from the outer aspect of the arms to the neck and nose, through the sinus passages, and down to the lungs and diaphragm, culminating in the large intestine. This explains the frequent correlation between respiratory and colon functional disturbances such as asthma and bowel dysfunctions. In acupuncture treatment of someone who suffers from asthma, sinusitis, and constipation, improvement in the bowel complaints or the sinus disorder may well occur before the asthma begins to improve. The patient may also become more aware of the dynamic interplay of the desire to be dependent coupled with a strong desire to remain separate. Bodymind-integrative acupuncture therapy will always treat the entire constellation of which asthma is only a part, rather than focus symptomatically on the asthma alone.

An acupuncturist may associate the Lung function with controlling Energy (Qi), circulating Blood, defense against external invaders, the nose and throat, the voice and the power of speech, the skin, the ability to take in and let go emotionally, grieving, and Life itself.

LUNG OBSTRUCTIONS

In addition to skin disorders such as eczema, which we looked at in Chapter 6, the forms of energetic disturbance affecting the Metal phase (Lung–Large Intestine) are multiple. Respiratory disorders include rhinitis, pharyngitis, laryngitis, bronchitis, asthma, and tuberculosis, which bespeak disturbances in the Lung meridian and energetic function and in the energy of the upper heater under the control of the Lungs. These disturbances are due to a deficiency of protective energy, especially in the fall and winter, when cold penetrates and injures these functions. Sinusitis and otitis may also occur through the associated Large Intestine energetic function, whose pathway traverses the ears and throat. Intestinal disturbances include predominantly left-sided colitis[17] with deficiency types of diarrhea and constipation, or heat in the intestines. Endocrine disorders may include hypothyroidism resulting from a deficiency of Sunlight Yang (Large Intestine and Stomach functions) and Greater Yin (Lung and Spleen functions), linked with a deficiency of the Yang transforming function of the Spleen and the Yang warming function of the Kidneys, leaving the body devoid of essential Fire and resulting in a slow metabolism. Pelvic complaints may arise owing to the trajectory of the Spleen meridian through the pelvic zones, and include scanty or absent menses (amenorrhea) due to a deficiency of Energy and Blood subsequent to a loss (grief is associated with Metal and the Lungs) or major worry (associated with Earth and Spleen).

Respiratory disturbances may also occur through energetic disturbances in other Elemental phases, especially those of Wood (Liver) and Water (Kidneys).

The major respiratory disturbances of the Wood phase are allergic asthma and hay fever (both aggravated by the pollen of spring), which occur suddenly like gusts of wind, indicative of the Wood phase. The major respiratory disturbances of the Water phase are stubborn, infectious disorders such as suppurative sinusitis, staphylococcus infection in the Lungs and throat, and acute or serious cases of tuberculosis of the Lungs, all due to a deficiency of the Yang of the Kidneys function, which brings into play adrenal activity, the stress response, and protective and immunological capacities; Kidney asthma, associated with an incident provoking great fear or fright, or an obstruction in the throat, often associated with a near drowning (fear of Water). In cases such as these, bodymind-integrative acupuncture therapy focuses not only on improving the function of the Upper Heater in general and the Lung function in particular, but also on the associated Wood or Water phases underlying the respiratory distress.

In treating a case of asthma associated with insomnia and a feeling of obstruction in the throat, in a patient who suffered a near drowning in childhood and had a deadly fear of water since, one would aim at alleviating the fear by tonifying the Kidney function (associated with fear and Water). Points on the lower back in the region of the Kidneys (on the second line of the Bladder meridian, which flows through this area), which are known for alleviating psychic blockage in the Kidney function, would be utilized, along with the opening points of the Conception Vessel and the Yin Heel Channel, which regulate the relationship between Metal (Lung 7) and Water (Kidney 6). One may also select points along the Kidney channel on the chest (Kidney 22–27) that are used in emotional disturbances of the Lungs or chest due to primary Kidney involvement, as well as Conception Vessel 22 in the throat, to open the throat zone. In my experience, such treatment quickly brings up the emotional issues associated with the near drowning (or, in some cases, with a perceived experience of the umbilical cord drawn taut around the unborn infant's throat), allowing for resolution of the core emotional as well as somatic blockages.

Just as sadness and grieving can prove injurious to Lung organ-energetic functioning in Five Phase energetics, leading to disorders of the skin as we saw in the previous chapter, we have observed that those suffering from Metal respiratory complaints are often prone to dark, depressive states. Such people often suffer from bronchitis or asthma as well as intestinal complaints precipitated by the loss of a loved one, where the separation is often associated with grieving that has not been vented. Acupuncture therapy in such instances will focus on the entire Metal phase imbalance.

Acupuncture therapy for respiratory complaints and weakness of the chest will focus on building the energy of the Upper Zone, promoting the free flow of protective energy and stimulating the Lung, Kidney, or Liver energetic functions, as the case may be, to increase respiratory activity, free up the diaphragm, and open the chest. This will lead to freer breathing, a sense of relief and the ability not only to take in more (physically and mentally), but also to let go, often accompanied by a crying spell. In this sense the blockage may well be seen as trapped tears leading to chest constriction.

AN ACHING HEART: CARDIAC FUNCTION, CIRCULATION, AND ANXIETY

In *Herz und Angst*, Ludwig Braun, a specialist in psychosomatic medicine, developed the concept of a "cardiac psyche" centered on anxiety, concluding that the heart is the "specific sense organ of anxiety."[18] Braun believed anxiety to be "an inner tactile sensation bound up with a special end apparatus, located in the cardiac tissue."[19] In acupuncture energetics this would involve not so much the Heart function as the Pericardium (Master of the Heart or Heart Protector) protective, armoring function as it works to create a muscular defense around the Heart to protect it against emotional trauma.

On the other hand, W. H. von Wyss, a contemporary of Braun, believed that the heart was "the organ of expression not only for anxiety, but for all affects."[20] Essentially, he believed that psychical processes resonate in the body just as somatic processes resonate in the psyche. In other words, "an affect contains not only its psychic experience, but also its motor expression to the outer world, and the resonance in the viscera, this latter representing a sort of language of the individual to himself"[21] and one of the most important organs of inner expression. Thus the Heart is intimately tied to the inner being of a person and, as in the Chinese portrayal, symbolizes the human spirit.

Thus it can be seen that the respiratory and cardiac functions of the Upper Zone together constitute the mainstay of Life, the cessation of either spelling the death of the individual. This is in keeping with the acupuncture-energetic view of the Lungs as responsible for circulating Energy, which in turn moves, oxygenates, and purifies the Blood. In addition, while the acupuncture-energetic physiological view portrays each organ-energetic function as storing some aspect of the psyche (*Shen*), it is the Heart, known as the "Supreme Controller," that oversees the workings of the bodymind.[22]

We shall now look at the heart from three different psychological perspectives: the classic psychosomatic concept of the heart or cardiac neurosis, a modern psychological view of migraine as a complex circulatory and bodymind disturbance, and the behavioral-psychological concept of the Type A personality.

A NERVOUS HEART

Dunbar, writing from the psychoanalytic-psychosomatic perspective, cites the paradoxical discovery that many patients suffering from actual organic heart disease show very little, if any, consciousness of their disease, and hence no insight into its meaning. Likewise, they tend to minimize their complaints, such as shortness of breath on exertion. "Heart neurotics," on the other hand, seem to suffer an intense subjective experience of heart or circulatory distress.[23] It may well be that one who takes note of physical weakness or stress points in the area of the heart, thereby generating a bodily awareness of even minor deviations in that function, is better able to divert stress away from the heart than the actual cardiac patient, who demonstrates an ignorance of body function that leaves the Heart unprotected, thereby exposing it to absorption of stress on a continual basis without an avenue of release. In acupuncture it is the Heart Protector (Master of the Heart) that is active in the "heart neurotic," whereas this function is deficient in the cardiac patient who, unable to protect his Heart against stress, succumbs in the cardiac zone.

The psychogenic factors most clearly associated with the Heart, according to Alexander, are free-floating anxiety and repressed rage. This corroborates the acupuncture-energetic perspective wherein the most common heart disorders tend to occur when there is a disturbance in the Water (Kidneys), Wood (Liver) and Fire (Heart) phases. For example, the fear and anxiety associated with a weakness of the Water phase will result in Water's inability to control Fire (the Heart), just as repressed rage will lead to constriction in the Liver (Wood) function, resulting in disturbed Heart (Fire) functions, since Wood is the mother of Fire.

Since the repressed hostility associated with this rage increases anxiety, these two emotional factors prove critical in the development of a cardiac neurosis. Alexander and Dunbar both conclude that with no prior organic disturbance, the heart may develop serious and even fatal conditions solely on the basis of psychic factors and events. They

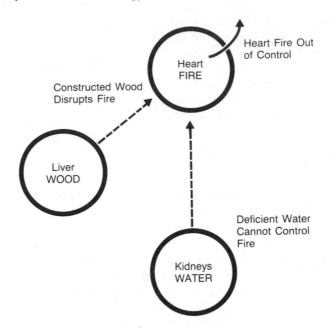

recommend the use of psychotherapy with these patients to make them aware of their bodymind imbalance. They emphasize that it is best not to allow such patients to dwell on either the psychological or the somatic components of their condition, while the practitioner must be aware of both.

The cardiac and circulatory disturbances most commonly studied from the classic psychosomatic perspective are essential hypertension and migraine.

Alexander shows that in the case of essential hypertension, there is a dynamic pattern beginning with fear and rage. As we saw in Chapter 4, one of the ways the bodymind prepares for fight or flight, by way of the sympathetic system, is through an increase in arterial tension, owing to the fact that the free expression of hostile drives has been largely prohibited. In a person who continuously reacts to situations with extreme inhibition of hostile drives, a chronic rise in blood pressure may occur owing to lack of an outlet for this rage.[24] In this instance, the bodymind is in a perpetual state of preparedness for fight or flight. It has been noted that often the hypertensive patient is one who was aggressive during childhood and suddenly shifted toward timidity in later years. As with the other organ-functional systems we have been discussing, psychodynamic factors are not sufficient in themselves to account for dysfunction, but act in combination with environmental factors and "still unknown, possibly inherited somatic factors."[25]

Migraine headache, according to Alexander, is often associated with repressed rage, sometimes against intellectually brilliant individuals, combined with a resentful attitude related to an inability to live up to perfectionistic tendencies. The common symptoms of migraine (periodicity of attack, paresthesia, speech difficulties, unilaterality to the pain, aversion to light, vomiting, and nausea, as well as a "marked sensation of well-being" after the attack) are sometimes reported to disappear in a matter of minutes, when given expression to in abusive words.[26]

THE MIGRAINE RESPONSE

In his authoritative work on the subject of migraine from a multidisciplinary perspective, Dr. Oliver Sacks, a noted neurologist, pointed out that migraine can occur without headache where the other common symptoms occur, along with "migraine aura," a kind of hallucinatory disturbance of the visual field. Concerning etiology, Sacks criticized the view of migraine as genetic, suggesting as more probable the environmental influence of the family and its own reaction patterns.[27] He also discredited any attempt to speak of a migraine constitutional type or "diathesis," unless this constitutional concept takes into account the multiplicity of possible factors and personality profiles involved. He made the interesting observation that migraine and allergic attacks are biologically analogous difficulties in adaptation.[28] In fact, Sacks's own experience with more than one thousand migraine patients implies that "the entire migraine may be perpetuated by one or another of its own symptoms. In short . . . *a migraine can become a response to itself.*"[29] Unlike other disorders, such as peptic ulcer, which can be shown to serve a particular emotional need, "migraines may be summoned to serve endless varieties of emotional needs," and patients' own theories of their causes will be as diverse as these needs, ascribing migraine attacks alternatively to intestinal complaints, menstruation, allergies, genes, stomach distress, or something they ate.[30] Therefore, he takes exception to the "stereotype of the obsessive migraine personality" or the existence in all migraine patients of "chronic repressed rage and hostility." He goes further in rejecting the notion of all migraine patients as neurotic (unless neurosis is seen as the human condition), "for in many cases . . . the migraines may replace a neurotic structure, constituting an alternative to neurotic desperation and assuagement."[31] Sacks leans toward the perspective of A. R. Luria, a Russian behaviorist, who sees physiological function as "a *functional system* directed toward the performance of a particular biological task . . . based on a 'dynamic constellation' of connections, situated at different levels of the nervous system . . . [which] may be freely substituted for one another or interchanged with the task remaining unchanged."[32]

This would account for the adaptation task or process having very different and changing mechanisms. This conclusion is far-reaching from a therapeutic perspective, for "*if migraine is necessary in the physiological or emotional economy of the individual, the attacks will continue to occur, to be elaborated, whatever particular mechanisms are eliminated.*"[33] As seen in Chapter 4, psychosomatic complexes are ongoing processes of life; as stated earlier, it may well prove salutary to have a somatic safety valve such as migraine in order to protect more important energetic and physiological functions.

Sacks concludes that the attempt to abort attacks with ergotamine or other such medications is extremely unwise. "One must work *with* one's biology, not against it; or one's biology will retaliate with a vengeance."[34] The best approach to migraine is self-help, in which the patient is guided, not treated, by the therapist or physician toward self-awareness and non-invasive therapies that prove effective for that particular patient. For, Sacks concludes, "It is not the migraine but the *patient* that needs treatment."[35] In keeping with what we have termed a bodymind-energetic approach, Sacks comments that "it is neither a technique nor a 'treatment' which the physician finally gives, though his giving must include techniques and treatments. What must finally be given is understanding—and courage: an *attitude* that is life-affirming in face of disease . . . [to] activate an inner power, a Healing Will."[36] This is reminiscent of Groddeck's concept that the "doctor's fate is to serve and to treat patients," not disease.[37] Groddeck said that the practitioner must put "his own psyche in the service of the patient, using his treatments—in all cases safe—as supporters of the patient's will to recover."[38]

It is unfortunate that Sacks, who clearly adheres to a phenomenological approach that attends to the moment of the person's real distress, and who has treated migraine sufferers for over fifteen years according to his own accounts, has not himself explored alternative techniques, such as acupuncture, bio-feedback, and other forms of stress reduction, since he recognizes in principle the value of such promising therapies. To adopt a broad phenomenological perspective focused on insight, without exploring effective and safe somatic therapies, shortchanges the client, as critics of psychoanalysis have long maintained. Psychological understanding and insight, while critical, must be combined with effective somatic treatments. The combination of insight and efficacious bodymind methods is clearly indicated in such conditions. What is powerful in Sacks's approach is the descriptive phenomenological method, aimed at describing, with patients, their own inner worlds in order to enable them to act to initiate their own healing.

Bernie Siegel, a surgeon with much experience in the treatment of cancer patients, uses a novel combination of counseling, art therapy, visualization, and surgery; emphasizes the need with such gravely ill patients to assess the strength of their wills to get well; and utilizes somatic and psychotherapeutic methods concurrently. Starting from an affirmation of life, Siegel asks patients to reflect back on important events that occurred in the year or two before their illness, often enabling them to pinpoint with great accuracy the psychic aspects of their somatic complaints. Siegel then asks his patients to reflect on the meaning of their illness and the need the illness fills. The result of this approach is that the patient is led, as in Sacks's approach, to take responsibility for the illness, which is the first step in assuming responsibility for initiating the necessary changes to bring about healing. Recognizing that all illness involves body and mind also means realizing that all successful therapy must involve both sides of the patient, in order to prod the will to recover.[39]

In this context, it is often crucial to make patients aware of their bodies, with which they have lost contact. "Many patients have lost contact with their physical selves, just as people sitting in a room with a clock grow so used to its ticking that they no longer hear it."[40]

TIME CONSTRAINTS AND CONSTRICTED ARTERIES

Friedman and Rosenman, behaviorists who developed the concept of Type A and Type B behavior (1974), cite an excess competitive drive and a chronic sense of time urgency as the two decisive characteristics of the Type A personality. Though usually able to control it, the Type A person may give way to short, apparently unwarranted outbursts of anger and hostility. Such a person is very impatient, suffering from "hurry sickness," and always has to be doing something, carrying out an activity he considers productive, so that no time is lost.[41] Time will be the enemy as this person sets deadlines that cannot be met. This sort of person judges things quantitatively, in terms of how much money and success are involved; does not have time for real leisure; is typically aggressive and outgoing; tends to focus on the present and his or her achievements only; and shows an inability to plan ahead, rarely stopping to ask what it all means. This person wants, above all else, to be respected by superiors and will sacrifice all to get this respect. Thus, the person's aggressivity will be taken out not on bosses, but on peers, as well as on close friends and loved ones. While this type of behavior has been tied to cardiovascular disease, a revised profile of the "coronary-prone individual" has been drawn up by Friedman and Rosenman. This profile is very different from the one just described, indicating that phlegmatic noncompetitive behavior and low self-esteem are major components of heart disease. This type of person, they maintain, overcompensates with Type A self-destructive behavior. "This driving orientation in an individual who is not of that inclination creates a profound stress and split in psychological orientation."[42] Friedman and Rosenman propose behavioral modification techniques in order to help a Type A personality learn non–Type A behavior, and they advise deep relaxation and meditation as well as attitude reorientation. While this research has led to a better understanding of some of the behavioral causes of heart disease, the fact is that such a simplified method of character typing often results in a fear-laden approach to these disorders that can create negative stress in and of itself. Information about the Type A personality was quickly disseminated by the media and resulted in a major increase in aerobic fitness programs for executives. Suddenly, everyone was certain of being a Type A person. People launched into supposedly beneficial cardiac fitness activity with the same stress-filled fervor that characterizes this personality type in the first place. Many have even become hooked on jogging or aerobic dance programs, and suffer rather severe mood swings if this activity must be curtailed. In short, it is possible that the over-simplified Type A profile was adopted by many non–Type A individuals.

A phenomenological bodymind approach would not assume a person's type as inevitably leading to a specific disease, but would work with the person to help promote awareness of his or her inner worlds, particular relationship to time, speed and duration of life, and relationship to space, both the space of the internal environment and the space of the outside world. In such an investigation with and on behalf of the patient, the person will discover in individual terms the constrictions in the bodymind, and the bodymind therapist will serve as a guide-educator, helping the person explore these constrictions in depth, in order to ascertain where they are localized and how they fit into the economy of his or her life. Body and mind therapies will be drawn on to enable the person to free up constricted zones. Acupuncture energetics will be of special importance, as the pattern depicted by the placement of needles will resonate with the once fully functional bodymind pattern that has been dysfunctional, thereby prodding the bodymind to recollect an aspect of being-in-the-world. Viewed in this light, acupuncture therapy is a bodymind integrative behavioral therapy, greatly enhanced when utilized with other behavioral therapies such as meditation, breathing and relaxation, self-hypnosis, and imaging.

ACUPUNCTURE ENERGETICS OF THE HEART

The energetic functioning of the Heart and Heart Protector functions, as we saw in Chapter 2, brings to mind the following acupuncture associations: cardiac and circulatory functions in general, the flow and control of the blood, the blood vessels, regulation of the heartbeat and pulse, the storehouse of the Spirit (*Shen*), rational behavior and a calm personality, the tongue and speech (and thus speech defects or fast speech), a reddish or pale complexion (lack of red, associated with the Fire phase); insomnia, restlessness, emotional warmth, and so forth.

Fire (Heart and Pericardium, or Heart Protector) energetic patterns are multiple, but the most common patterns include the following:

• Vascular spasms and high blood pressure, often combined with Liver-energetic hyperactivity in which the "Rising Liver Fire" agitates its child, the Heart, leading to "Heart Fire Blazing Upward" with disturbed cardiac function, a red complexion, agitation, fast or slurred speech, "hurry sickness" characteristic of the Type A profile, and tightness in the chest;

• Pins and needles or achiness along the pathways of the Heart and Pericardium meridians, on the inner aspect of the palms and arms to the armpit and chest;

• Disturbances of the arteries and veins due to congealed (stuck) Blood from a deficiency of Blood or Energy in these energetic functions;

• Swollen ankles (around the Kidney meridian zone, since the Kidney-Water is the lower branch of Lesser Yin, of which the Heart-Fire meridian is the upper branch);

• Disorders of the Small Intestine, as the Heart, when agitated, will attempt to dump the excess heat into its Yang-paired bowel, namely the Small Intestine meridian;

• Emotional disturbances affecting the strength of the personality as a whole, since the Heart rules the bodymind, such as general weakness and lethargy associated with depression, loss of memory (as the Heart, thus weakened, cannot feed its child, the Spleen, the latter governing memory and concentration), hysteria, emotional extremes, general agitation and nervousness, anxiety with an absence of laughter in the voice, and a lack of Fire in the complexion and the personality, or "false" laughter.

Cardiac and circulatory disturbances and patterns can result from primary disturbances in other elemental energetic functions as well.

If the Wood (Liver) is in excess, the Heart will grow agitated, with migraines; red, irritated eye disorders; heart palpitations; and precordial pain. This will bring into play the pathway of the Pericardium (Hand Absolute Yin) meridian, coupled with the Liver (Foot Absolute Yin), often associated with cardiac neuroses and panic syndromes. If the Water (Kidney) is deficient, it will not be able to properly control Fire (Heart and Pericardium) along the normal control cycle of the Five Elements, resulting in a loss of harmony between Water and Fire with low backache, loss of sexual Fire, achiness in the knees, possible hearing disorders, dizziness, emotional outbursts, insomnia, and an ever-present fear.

Treatment of the Heart- or Heart Protector-energetic functions must focus either on calming Heart Fire, in the case of hyperactivity, with such points as the Spirit Gate, Heart 7, and the back points associated with Heart and Pericardium functional and psychological aspects (namely points on the Bladder meridian over the region of the Heart and Pericardium, and points along the midline in the front known as Alarm points for these two functions), or strengthening the energy of the Heart, by tonifying its "mother," the Liver, as well as the Heart and Pericardium directly.

In disorders of Heart function involving other energetic phases, such as Water or Wood as in the examples just given, the primary focus will be on treating the Water (Kidney) or Wood (Liver) directly, with secondary focus on the Heart or Pericardium functions. Treatment will also aim at restoring the normal energetic cycles of control or generation between Water, Wood, and Fire functions. In my experience the images of Water (Moisture, Fluidity) and Fire (Dryness, Heat) prove especially useful in prodding a recollection on the part of a patient suffering from disorders affecting the psyche or the spirit.

In his attempt to move analytical (Jungian) psychology out of the purely psychic realm to include the reality of the body, physical illness, and the material decomposition of death, Dr. Alfred Ziegler, a Swiss Jungian analyst and physician specializing in psychosomatic medicine, developed an approach akin to the bodymind-energetic approach that he termed "archetypal medicine."

In this method, the physician focuses on the subjective reality of the patient's own worlds, and aims at providing a phenomenological amplification of archetypal images that arise in the therapeutic process, especially where these images "carry the symbolic essence and are accompanied by perceptible physical resonance."[43] This sort of practitioner works less like a scientist focused on "objective" details and more like a "poet who muses" on "the art of interpreting primal images."[44]

Like the behavioral acupuncture and bodymind-energetic approaches we have been discussing, archetypal medicine focuses not on disease units per se, but rather on patterns, "more or less reversible, mutable syndromes (images of illness)."[45] These patterns often appear as a dynamic interplay of opposite forces, at times achieving a special harmony and at other times distorted to the point of a body/mind split resulting in somatization.

The above-mentioned opposition appears frequently between Water and Fire: between an extreme of fluidity, which would end in loss or drowning in the formless Sea, to be countered by Fire and dryness, by calling up images of what is pure, "through which everything arises out of the flood of the indistinguishable";[46] and between an extreme of dryness, returning everything back to dust and nothingness, countered by moisture, fluidity, and the wavelike forces of water as it moves through the bodymind.

Drying, burning, wasting Fire conditions are due to a deficiency of the Water Root of life (Deficient Yin, especially in the Kidneys), where the lack of moisture results in a fast metabolism, with a tendency toward hyperthyroidism or hypertension, dryness, agitation, and a disturbed spirit. Images of Water, of moisture, of the forces of the Moon working especially at night to moisten the bodymind and restore the primacy of fluid metabolism in the organism will be especially suited for patients suffering these "becoming-hot" patterns, such as high blood pressure, insomnia, nervousness, agitated speech, and general shakiness of the spirit. Bodymind energetic therapy for these people must focus on strengthening and increasing Water in the body and fluidity in the psyche, in order to control the "false Fire" that would ultimately consume them.

In those suffering from a deficiency of the Fire Root, on the other hand (especially Fire or Yang of the Kidneys), there will occur patterns of uncontrolled fluid accumulation, as in congestive heart failure with fluid around the heart, or all manner of edematous disorders. Such people will show a lack of emotional warmth, and a deficiency of body heat, and will have a feeling of emotional and physical coldness and moistness. Their patterns will portray a becoming-cold and becoming-moist tendency, with leanings toward hypothyroidism and low blood pressure, a build-up of coldness and dampness (mucus and edema) in the body, and general lethargy and sluggishness in their behavior and demeanor. Images of Fire, of an increase in the forces of heat in the body, through the action of the Sun as it burns down on and warms the organism, will be of special benefit to these people, and bodymind energetic therapy in this case will focus on combatting an uncontrolled accumulation of fluids, dampness, and cold in the body by increasing the Fire Root to warm the body and promote emotional warmth and a capacity for Joy (associated, through the Five Element theory, with the Fire Element and the Heart) in the psyche, in order to prevent Water from overcoming and drowning them.

In helping patients engage in a dialogue and encounter with images of internal metabolism, of Water and Fire, "a philosophical standpoint obtrudes upon us and requires of both physician and patient a contemplation of the archetypal in fluids and in dry things . . . as if we, despite all the therapy, would not otherwise know where we stand."[47] This leads patient and therapist alike toward a *virtual center*, different for each person, present within the very center of that person's being-in-the-present. This is the phenomenological practitioner's own particular standpoint, from which a genuine therapeutic encounter may emerge.

A CASE OF PANIC IN THE UPPER ZONE

From a bodymind-energetic perspective an understanding of complaints of the Upper Zone (Heart and Lung energetic functions) must derive from a detailed investigation of the emotional, psychological, and spiritual issues involved, as well as from a careful scrutiny of the somatic-energetic zones and reaction patterns displayed. In the following case, acupuncture energetics and bodymind-integrative use of imaging techniques will be shown to enhance each other's effects.

I have recently begun work that holds the promise of creating an imaginal acupuncture. It involves combining acupuncture therapy and imaging techniques by drawing on the images and metaphors of acupuncture energetics. I first initiated this project under the guidance of Dr. Gerald Epstein, a New York–based psychiatrist specializing in bodymind-integrative therapy that he terms "waking dream therapy."[48] If acupuncture treatment can help a person gain a bodily felt sense of improved functioning, then imaging techniques aimed at consolidating the acupuncture treatment by guiding the patient to administer imaginal acupuncture should theoretically make it possible to reduce the number of acupuncture sessions involved and enable the patient to take more control of the healing process, making use of the acupuncture therapist only when necessary.

The following case will illustrate this approach. This patient was a senior student completing a master's degree in business at a prestigious university. As a top student he expected, upon graduation, to receive the job of his choice in a highly competitive and lucrative profession.

The young man was suffering from a series of vague but highly distressing complaints, centered on what had been tentatively diagnosed by one psychologist as panic syndrome. He was not interested in taking the medications usually prescribed for this condition, and intensive psychotherapy had been of only minimal help in abating the physical symptoms. These included agitated sleep, irritability, constant anxiety, tightness of the musculature throughout the body, and fatigue.

Appearing calm on the surface, the patient grew visibly anxious as soon as I began to take his pulse and comment on the high level of constriction I felt in his body (as indicated by a wiry, thin, tight pulse). His legs started to shake uncontrollably. I mentioned that in someone with as much internal tension as I perceived him to have, such shaking fits were virtually unavoidable and allowed some outlet for the tension. He then began to talk about his upcoming career in the stressful world of investment banking and noted that while he was an excellent student who could land any job he wished, he did not feel that such high-stress work was for him.

At this point I explained the stress response in behavioral and acupuncture-energetic terms, as a way of providing him with metaphors that I hoped would stir up images of his disorder and his dilemma. We talked about the way the adrenals (the Fire of the Kidneys), the musculature (under the control of the Liver, and agitated by repressed anger), the blood vessels, and the heart pump itself gear up when a perceived threat arises, preparing the bodymind for fight or flight. He commented that this description rang true and brought together into one picture all his concerns and complaints.

I explained that under normal circumstances, after the fight had been waged or the organism had retreated from the danger that had brought into play the sympathetic nervous system, there would be a vegetative retreat to the parasympathetic functions of resting and digesting, in order for the bodymind to replenish itself. In the high-pressured urban world, especially the one he was planning to enter, the fight or flight is never concluded but is ongoing, leading to chronic stress without the resulting parasympathetic reprieve.

In acupuncture energetics this prompts the Liver (Wood), filled with repressed rage at not being able to be freely creative and expressive in the outside world, to invade the Spleen (Earth), resulting in gastric, often pre-ulcerous constriction in the pit of the stomach and a longing for motherly love and nourishment. At this moment the patient grew teary-eyed and "admitted," as he put it, that he had long ago foregone any hope of possessing a mother or a father, since his parents had never understood who he really was. Pressure from his family to become financially successful and independent had forced him to train for a lucrative career and draw on his competitive nature, to the detriment of his sensitive and intellectual character, which drew him in the direction of philosophy or literature.

He described his mother as emotional and volatile, always focused on her own needs and not at all loving or giving. His father was absent and detached, a non-entity in his life.

At this point he commented that his relationship with women had always been strained and would rarely last more than a few months, although women were easily attracted to him and he "never had to work at finding a girlfriend."

I spoke to him about the Water Phase (Kidney), which in his case was frozen by fear and anxiety, as demonstrated by a slow, almost absent pulse in the third position on his right wrist—the position associated with the Fire of the Kidney (*and* the Heart Protector), which under normal conditions would be in a harmonious, checking relationship with the Fire Phase (Heart and Pericardium) and would nourish the Wood (Liver) Phase. I asked him to lie on the table on his back, so that I could palpate his body to find sensitive or constricted zones. I began to palpate, conscientiously, the zones under discussion: the pit of the stomach and the diaphragm, up through the chest to the throat. Constriction in the Liver pathway was evident since the deficient Water was not nourishing its child, Wood; this was leading to an inability for Wood to nourish its child, the Heart, leaving the Heart uncontrolled (Water, being weak, cannot control Fire), and obliging the Heart Protector to work excessively, to exhaustion, to protect the heart against external stressors. Palpation revealed the most constricted body I had encountered in ten years of acupuncture work. With the mildest pressure on any points along the affected zones, his body would shake uncontrollably, and he would at times laugh, or almost cry, but implore me not to stop. He was impressed at how easily the acupuncture evaluation had led to precisely the areas of his tension. I used the occasion to explain to him that tightness in the area a few inches above his navel, in the absence of an ulcer, aneurysm, or intestinal obstruction, would be doubtless dismissed by an internist as nothing to worry about. In my own understanding of his body/mind split, I explained, what had been diagnosed as panic syndrome started in the pit of his stomach, owing to a weakness and coldness in his pelvic zone (the region of Kidney Energy). I had him feel the coldness below his navel, and the hard rod running from a few inches above his navel all the way up to his sternum, as well as the constriction in his throat. This tracing of the relevant energetic zones has become very important in my way of practicing a bodymind-integrative acupuncture therapy, as it sets the stage for a recollection of forgotten energetic pathways that I hope to stimulate in the acupuncture treatment. The patient speculated that his Heart-Fire was burning so low because of his frozen Kidney-Fire, and added that in his relationships with women he felt both this frozenness in his sexual center and lack of warmth in his heart. I asked him if he thought this might be due to the overactive Heart Protector, which was building a muscular wall around his chest and preventing any intense feelings from coming in or out. He said that was exactly what was happening in his life.

He expressed some fear about the insertion of needles, as he felt the acupuncture evaluative process itself had unveiled so much that he was afraid the needling would leave him totally vulnerable. I assured him that the needling would be far more stabilizing than my clumsy attempt at explanation, as words were always full of errors and inaccuracies that could lead to confusion, while acupuncture therapy itself, when practiced carefully, was a purely phenomenological process attuned to the patient's present state of being. I explained that I would be needling a pattern of points to help his bodymind remember how to function in the Kidney zone, thereby moistening the Liver, allowing the musculature to relax and the energy now trapped in his diaphragm (which classic psychosomaticians would have diagnosed as a diaphragmatic neurosis) to flow evenly up to his chest, calming the Heart Protector and easing the Spirit and the Mind. I said this while asking him to practice relaxed breathing focused on bringing the breath down to the center of his diaphragmatic knot, pacing my comments to his breathing, then slowing my speech down (utilizing the simple pacing-and-leading techniques of Ericksonian hypnotherapy) to help lead him to a more relaxed state. I then needled the following constellation of points, which I trusted would resonate with his current state: Liver 5 and Pericardium 5, to treat the underlying Absolute Yin somatic energetic reaction pattern of constriction and free up the diaphragm zone; Pericardium 1, on the sides of the chest; Liver 14, beneath the nipples; Kidney 23, on the chest; and Conception Vessel 17, in the center of the Chest. All had been exquisitely sensitive in the physical examination. I pressed with firm pressure first, before needling, to prime the body for the needling reaction I was seeking. I then needled Conception Vessel 10, a few inches above the navel on his midline, explaining that his breathing should flow there, freeing up the constriction and opening the diaphragm and chest. I ended with Kidney 2 and 3, the Fire and Source points of the Kidney meridian, respectively, to build the Kidney's Fire Root and help rid his bodymind of "chilling fear." I then instructed him to continue the breathing, and while closing his eyes to imagine the feeling, texture, sound, color, odor, or image of what was constricted in his diaphragm. If he arrived at an image of a knot, he was to untie it; if of a hard ball, he was to allow it to turn to wax and melt; and so forth. I then left him alone for about ten minutes.

When I returned he said he had been crying, but was now very peaceful, almost asleep, and felt as if he were floating above the table. I noted that the pulse was no longer wiry and tight, and mentioned to him that it now felt as though a free flow of water were coursing through his body. He remarked that that was exactly what he had imagined while lying there. I palpated his stomach and the knot was greatly reduced. I had him verify this, explaining that whenever he felt tension developing in his body, he was to go off alone for a moment, place his fingers on this spot, close his eyes, and remember the way he had just now restored a free flow of fluidity to his body. I also had him feel his pelvic zone, which had warmed up markedly, and his chest, which was smooth, relaxed, and virtually spasm-free.

At the second session, the patient reported he had been much less tense that week and was able to ease tension whenever it began with simple exercises of relaxed breathing and imaging along with pressure on the tight area in his stomach. He felt as if his "Heart Protector were easing up a bit, to allow genuine feelings of love and warmth to flood [his] body." He felt greatly energized but at the same time calm, a state he had previously thought impossible.

This way of practicing acupuncture therapy, combined with behavioral and psychosomatic understanding and techniques, has led me to reduce by over half the number of sessions needed by most patients and to allow far longer intervals between sessions after the first few treatments. I have found that bodymind practices such as acupuncture can become very addictive, and I work carefully to prevent patients from becoming dependent on me or on the therapy, placing them in the center of their own healing process armed with new self-therapeutic skills.

I am aware that some practitioners or critics of bodymind approaches will read the above case as proof that acupuncture works by suggestion or placebo. It is even conceivable that some acupuncturists, holding to the modern Chinese view of acupuncture as merely a physical therapy, will feel critical of the use of Western relaxation, suggestion, and pacing-and-leading techniques during the counseling and palpation phase of treatment, and will view imaging techniques as alien to true Chinese acupuncture. Purists—deluded, I think, by the belief that clinical practice must be guided by the scientific method—will criticize this combination of therapies, claiming that it clouds the treatment and renders it impossible to know if the acupuncture (and if so, which of the acupuncture points) was effective.

As a clinician I assume that the effect of any therapy is a result of the combined use of the therapeutic techniques themselves and the use the therapist makes of his or her own person, to create a resonance in the patient that catalyzes meaningful transformation.

K. C. Cole, writing on physics in everyday life, stresses the fact that when we speak of being on the same wavelength as someone else, we are speaking as scientifically as a pure physicist does when speaking of resonance in the universe. *Resonance,* the aim of bodymind energetic work, means to resound or echo, as in a *sympathetic vibration* with another human being or with the cosmos. Cole defines the force of resonance thus: "the power of resonance comes literally from being in the right place at the right time. For it to work, there has to be a harmony between what you're doing and the way something (or someone) wants to go . . . . Resonance, in other words, allows a lot of little pushes in the right place to add up to big results."[49] I like to conceive of the placement of acupuncture needles in a particular constellation or configuration as "a well-timed kick in the pants."[50] The placement of needles, the use of images, and the prodding of the patient's own imaginal experiences are all so many little pushes, guided by a clear intention on the part of the practitioner of the bodymind-energetic approach, that serve as a catalyst to promote change by prodding the bodymind to heal itself in its own way.

NOTES

1. As paraphrased from G. R. Heyer, in Flanders Dunbar, *Emotions and Bodily Changes,* p. 237.
2. Cf. Kaptchuk, *The Web That Has No Weaver,* p. 69.
3. Cf. Pelletier, *Mind as Healer, Mind as Slayer,* p. 23.
4. Dunbar, *Emotions and Bodily Changes,* p. 242.
5. Ibid., p. 238.
6. Dunbar, p. 240.
7. Alexander, *Psychosomatic Medicine,* p. 133.
8. Ibid., p. 134.
9. Cf. Margaret W. Gerard, "Bronchial Asthma in Children" in Franz Alexander and Morton French, *Studies in Psychosomatic Medicine.* New York, Ronald Press, 1943, p. 243.
10. Ibid., p. 245.
11. Ibid., pp. 245; 259–262.
12. Groddeck, *The Meaning of Illness,* p. 125.
13. For similar exercises to treat respiratory complaints, Cf. Gerald Epstein, *Waking Dream Therapy.* New York, Human Sciences Press, 1981.
14. Alexander, *Psychosomatic Medicine,* p. 134.
15. Cf. Ibid., p. 135.
16. Ibid., p. 139.
17. Cf. Yves Requena, *Terrains and Pathology in Acupuncture.* Brookline, Massachusetts, Paradigm Publications, 1986, on the YangMing (Sunlight Yang) temperament; and Kiko Matsumoto, on the Deficient Liver/Large Intestine Excess abdominal confirmation in unpublished teachings, New England School of Acupuncture, 1985–86.

18. As quoted in Dunbar, *Emotions and Bodily Changes,* p. 206.
19. Ibid., p. 207.
20. As quoted by Dunbar, p. 207.
21. Ibid.
22. Cf. Dianne Connelley, *Traditional Acupuncture: Law of the Five Elements,* Chapter on the Fire function. Centre for Traditional Acupuncture, p. 45.
23. Dunbar, *Emotions and Bodily Changes,* p. 208.
24. Alexander, *Psychosomatic Medicine,* p. 149.
25. Ibid., p. 149.
26. Ibid. pp. 157–160.
27. Oliver Sacks, M.D., *Migraine: Understanding a Common Disorder.* Berkeley, University of California Press, 1985, pp. 59–60; 132–134.
28. Ibid., pp. 172–173.
29. Ibid., p. 174.
30. Ibid., p. 180.
31. Ibid., p. 177.
32. Ibid., pp. 195–196.
33. Ibid., p. 196.
34. Ibid., pp. 223–224.
35. Ibid., p. 231.
36. Ibid.
37. G. Groddeck, *The Meaning of Illness,* p. 211.
38. Ibid.
39. Bernie S. Siegel, M.D., *Love, Medicine and Miracles: Lessons Learned About Self-Healing From a Surgeon's Experience With Exceptional Patients.* New York, Harper & Row, 1986, pp. 105–112.
40. Ibid., p. 140.
41. Cf. Pelletier, *Mind as Healer, Mind as Slayer,* pp. 125–126.
42. Ibid., p. 129.
43. Alfred J. Ziegler, M.D., *Archetypal Medicine,* translated from the German by Gary V. Hartman. Dallas, Texas, Spring Publications, Inc., 1983, p. 3.
44. Ibid., pp. 154–155.
45. Ibid., p. 159.
46. Ibid., pp. 161–162.
47. Ibid., p. 167.
48. Cf. Gerald Epstein, *Waking Dream Therapy,* cited previously. This work is being carried out with my colleague, Fay Jean Knell, an art therapist and acupuncturist, in our joint project for a Meridian Energetics Coloring Book.
49. K. C. Cole, *Sympathetic Vibrations.* New York, Bantam Books, 1985, pp. 265–266.
50. Ibid., p. 266.

8

Phenomenology of the Middle Zone: Giving, Receiving, and Gastrointestinal Complaints

An emotional disturbance affecting the alimentary canal is capable of starting a vicious circle . . . . Just as feelings of comfort and peace of mind are fundamental to normal digestion, so discomfort and mental discord may be fundamental to disturbed digestion.[1]

W. B. Cannon

There are striking parallels between the classic psychosomatic and acupuncture-energetic conceptualizations of the stomach and intestinal organ functions. The Stomach and Spleen-Pancreas functions, related to the Earth Phase in acupuncture, are concerned with issues of orality, receiving, and taking and giving nourishment, while the Large Intestine function, related to the Metal Phase in acupuncture, brings into play issues centered on anality, giving, expelling, and separating from the mother (Earth).

For purposes of discussion we shall separate gastric from intestinal functions and complaints in order to underscore the relationship between orality and the Earth Element, and between anality and the Metal Element in acupuncture energetics.

GATEWAY TO THE SOUL

As we saw in Chapters 2 and 3, the Stomach and Spleen Officials, related to the Earth Element, are disturbed directly in their functioning by worry and anxious doubt, and indirectly by grief, which injures their child Metal functions (Lung and Large Intestine), thereby draining their mother, Earth, functions. Likewise, the Earth functions may be invaded by overactive Wood (Liver and Gallbladder) functions, if the latter are agitated by anger, repressed rage, or other volatile emotions, by way of the Five Phase destruction cycle. Cannon, a specialist in psychosomatics, noted in his discussion of gastric disorders precisely the same emotions the ancient Chinese practitioners did as contributing factors in gastric complaints, and highlighted the "importance of avoiding so far as possible the initial states of worry and anxiety, and of not permitting grief and anger and other violent emotions to prevail unduly."[2]

Naturally, the pathway to the stomach, in Eastern and Western formulations, is the mouth, which has always played a significant part in myths and legends of humanity's inner turmoil. In many traditional cultures the main pathway for escape of the soul was thought to be through the mouth; in some traditional cultures the nose and mouth are covered to prevent the soul's escape.[3] The movements of the mouth, as Grinker, a noted psychiatrist, tells us, begin at the fourteenth fetal week.[4] At birth sucking is immediately functional, and at eight weeks the infant opens the mouth in anticipation of the nipple. At twelve weeks the child can purse the lips, and by twenty weeks the lower lip is capable of becoming activated and drawing in on a spoon as it is removed. Chewing, with the appearance of the teeth, follows. By three months of age the infant also begins hand–mouth interaction, with the resultant autoerotic pleasures and the beginning of the body-ego.

Sucking obviously provides the infant with pleasure above and beyond nutrition. Biting, itself, is also pleasurable, and survives in adulthood in the pleasure of eating, drinking, and chewing. According to psychoanalytic literature, oral pleasures are often a preliminary to genital satisfaction. Thus, if there are early oral disappointments, the object of desire is devoured, incorporated, and preserved in the psyche, leading to oral sadism.

As seen in Chapter 2, the beginnings of the body-ego are rooted in internal bodily sensations of physiological functioning.

Melanie Klein, the celebrated child psychoanalyst, postulated that initial oral frustration leads to sadism with fantasies of devouring and introjecting the good and bad parts of the mother's body, followed by efforts to expel them. Therefore, swallowing and regurgitation are energetic phenomena laden with psychic symbolism. The oral phase is sometimes defined in the psychosomatic literature as the wish to be devoured, to devour, and then to sleep (parasympathetic functioning, based on memories of nursing).[5]

One swallows and incorporates the outer world into the inner world of the stomach.[6] These two worlds come together, as we saw in Chapter 4, in the "oral cavity" created by the mother's cradling arms, breast, and flesh, and the infant's receptive mouth. Oral satiation leads to digestive peace and vice versa.

The classic psychosomatic perspective, then, sees the mouth as the pathway for the maintenance of life itself, a source of sensual satisfaction and a way of aggressively mastering reality (by biting, chewing, devouring, and absorbing it and its powers). Therefore, the psychoanalytic concepts of introjection, incorporation, and projection are intimately connected to the physiological functions of sucking, biting, digesting, and vomiting. The most prominent eating disorders linked to the oral stage, anorexia and bulimia, are related to the desire to store and retain, or on the other hand eliminate, food equivalent to the Mother, linked with guilt and depression.[7]

The infant's first need, after air (as we saw in Chapter 7), is for food. Satisfaction of this need leads to a primary release of tension and to sleep. Therefore, satiation is inextricably bound to one's developing sense of being nourished and loved, and if these needs are not met by "adequate mothering" (Winnicott), frustration, fear, and rage will develop. This, in turn, may lead to an overpowering anxiety.

The key to the oral stage is the mother–child dyad. At the end of the oral stage (Earth), the child separates from the mother and becomes a self-proclaimed individual (separation-individuation). This separation includes introjection of the "good" and "bad mothers," and development of the super-ego, generating a sense of shame and anxiety in the child. The anal stage (Metal functions), already begun by this point, will involve expelling and projecting, or retaining.

Any issue involving loss of an important object or loved one, or inability to solve a real problem, brings into play the child–mother, mouth–nipple psychosomatic pattern. This pattern revolves around deep disappointment leading to incomplete or inadequate separation from the mother, or other source of nourishment and love, and a resultant inability or difficulty in forming relationships.

Grinker believes, along with many other psychosomaticians, that problems associated with mothering are more specifically *somatic* in nature than those involving the father, harkening back as they do to the oral stage. Therefore, the mother–child dyad serves as the matrix for development of psychosomatic disorders. "All inner processes enter into transactional relationships with the environment at the surfaces of the body where they can be experienced. The biological and psychological organization of infant and mother and what goes on between them at all surfaces needs extensive research."[8]

ENERGY ACCUMULATIONS AND THE WISH TO BE FED

Franz Alexander describes the oral stage in somewhat more energetic terms. The infant's first concern is to accumulate and retain energy,[9] since its main activity is growth. Rapid growth during the first few months of life, accompanied by helpless dependency, leads to a dominant preoccupation with nourishment and being taken care of and loved.

For Freud, pleasure in the oral-energetic zone created by sucking and the dependent, passive, receptive, and demanding attitudes related to the mother are central in this stage. Therefore, sucking relates to receptive and incorporative drives. But when the flow of milk is insufficient, the child bites to get more, with this oral aggressivity following on the primary oral receptiveness. This early oral tendency, according to Freud, is possessive and connected to envy.

This most central concern of early life, namely eating/nursing/satiation, leads to a sense of satisfaction and well-being. The fear of starvation, on the other hand, is related to insecurity. According to Alexander, the most significant emotional dynamics present in all alimentary disturbances, then, are possessiveness, greed, jealousy, envy, and a striving for security. When more mature genital functions are disturbed, with inhibition due to psychic conflicts, emotional disturbances revolving around nutrition and orality may crop up.

In surveying the chief psychosomatic complaints of digestion, we see associations on the one hand between nervous vomiting and the expelling of what had been incorporated psychically, and on the other hand between swallowing and the inability or refusal to incorporate some material, laden with psychic significance.

In the case of gastric neuroses themselves, Alexander states, it is very difficult to differentiate between nervous and organic factors. In such instances, the multiplicity of factors involved are identical to those stressed in the Chinese medical literature: faulty eating habits, such as incomplete chewing, eating fast, swallowing air, overeating, eating poor food, and eating when emotionally upset. Hypoacidity, on the other hand, is related to depression. Schindler noted that hyposecretion of gastric juices "is one of the most important somatic symptoms of psychoneurotic depression," and designated this syndrome, remarkably similar to acupuncture patterns of deficiency of the Spleen Qi (which holds up the organs and promotes normal digestion) thus: *anacidity accompanied by ptosis and atonic constipation, the gastrointestinal correlate of depression.*[10]

Hyperacidity is related to the same emotional conflicts as peptic ulcer. In such conditions, there appears to be a fixation in early dependent situations that is in conflict with the adult sense of self, resulting in hurt pride. The ensuing wish for dependence, Alexander maintains, must be repressed, leading to development of intense gastric conflict, and ultimately to an ulcer. The common denominator in most gastric complaints, Alexander concludes, is a longing for reprieve, rest, help, and security (parasympathetic longings). Vacations often prove of great benefit in such cases, as they take attention off the core symptoms. It is critical in these disorders to focus as little as possible on the nature of the symptoms themselves, as this leads only to their exacerbation, but to place attention instead on the meaning of the symptoms, which must be understood in order for the core of the complex to be resolved.

The great success of acupuncture-energetic therapy in most gastrointestinal disorders is due, in no small measure, to the possibility of stimulating more appropriate gastric activity by locating the core somatic-energetic reaction pattern involved and selecting a configuration of points that resonates with this core pattern, without intellectual discussion of the symptoms. After a brief explanation of the acupuncture energetics of the middle zone, and palpation of this zone to help the patient gain a bodily sense of the imbalances, needling the appropriate set of points will prod a deep recognition by the patient of the underlying meaning of the gastric distress. This often results in a dramatic reduction of the gastric symptoms. The long-lasting effects of acupuncture-energetic therapy in such cases is due to its ability to prod precise energetic functions *in the body*, with insight following upon this bodily felt understanding.

The type of person who often develops peptic ulcers, Alexander and his colleagues observed, is the aggressive executive, who frequently rejects the softer, more nourishing feminine tendencies in his own nature (thereby rejecting, from an acupuncture-energetic perspective, his Earth center). More important than the personality configuration of the peptic ulcer patient, however, is the nature of the conflicts involved. The wish to be cared for and loved is in conflict with the wish to be totally independent. Persons battling such a conflict often show exaggerated aggressivity, great ambition, an independent air, and a tendency to assume responsibilities rather than accept help. Just as common, though, are patients who are overtly dependent. In such cases the conflict arises from external rather than internal circumstances, which frustrate the possibility of satisfying these dependent wishes. The crucial factor in either case is a primary frustration of dependent desires revolving around a demand for help and love, leading to stepped-up gastric activity and frustrated oral cravings.

"If the wish to receive, to be loved, to depend on others is rejected by the adult ego," Alexander concludes, "or frustrated through external circumstances and consequently cannot find gratification in personal contacts, then often a regressive pathway is used: the wish to be loved becomes converted into the wish to be fed."[11] This in turn mobilizes stomach innervations and leads to chronic stimulation of gastric functions, with resultant gastric dysfunctions down the road. In such instances, the stomach responds continuously as if food, love, and the mother were about to be received. The person suffering from a nervous stomach attests to this chronic sensation of an "empty middle," an *unloved Self*. Often there will be a secretion of gastric juices in such cases, especially at night. It is therefore advisable that some sort of totally relaxing activity be engaged in before retiring, such as a brisk walk, meditation, or relaxation techniques.

In some patients suffering gastric distress, especially some forms of anorexia, Ziegler, a Jungian analyst and psychosomatic physician, noticed a "compulsion to avoid succumbing to the sluggishness and inertia of the gravitational pull of all that is earthly."[12]

In these patients, Alexander and his colleagues found that there is often a constitutional weakness, or early acquired disturbance, in the Stomach function itself, which they believed had to be treated somatically. Here again, acupuncture-energetic therapy will be of great use in breaking or preventing a somatic compliance in the middle zone, thereby hastening resolution of the core issues involved.

THE ACUPUNCTURE ENERGETICS OF ORALITY

From an acupuncture-energetic perspective, the mouth calls to mind the Earth-organ functions of Stomach and Spleen, the Extra meridian Chungmo (Thrusting Channel), which traverses the gastric functions and connects with the Spleen function internally, all of which energize the base of the tongue, the gastrointestinal tract, and the ability to articulate freely.

The process of digestion in acupuncture energetics consists of the incorporation of energy from food combined with Air (Qi) to form the body's "nourishing energy" (*jing qi*). The digestive zone is also considered to be the barrier that separates and unites inside and outside.

Digestive disturbances will involve all of the Organ functions of the Middle Zone, namely the Wood (Liver and Gallbladder) and Earth (Spleen and Stomach) functions. Disturbances will often involve worry or fatigue, which together injure the Yang of the Spleen, making it unable to properly digest food. This deficiency may lead to hyperactivity and hyperacidity ("heat") in the Stomach function, or to increased activity in the Liver and Gallbladder functions, which will then invade the Earth functions along the destruction cycle of the Five Phases.

ACUPUNCTURE PATTERNS OF
DIGESTIVE DISTRESS

When the Spleen (Foot Greater Yin), connected with the Lung, (Hand Greater Yin channel) is disturbed, Stomach functioning will immediately be disturbed. In an excess of the Spleen function, there will be a slowing down of its ability to transform, leading to malabsorption, gas, and constipation. When there is a deficiency of Spleen functioning, there will be loose stools with undigested food particles. Belching and vomiting are clear signs of Spleen deficiency, attesting to an accumulation of Stomach "heat" that quickly ascends straight up the esophagus or by way of the extra connecting vessel from the point just below the nipple (Stomach 18) to the heart, with accompanying heartburn (the *Xu Li* vessel). In such cases the body will feel heavy, since the Spleen controls the extremities, and lack of this function leads to dampness and a bogged-down feeling. Abdominal swelling is a common symptom of the Spleen and the Small Intestine functions (Small Intestine–Fire is the "mother" of the Yang of the Spleen-Earth). Finally, a common symptom of Spleen deficiency, owing to the Spleen meridian's connection to the Lung meridian, is hiccuping.

Loss of appetite and indigestion frequently occur in patterns of Spleen dysfunction. Chinese texts emphasize, as does the psychosomatic literature, that proper eating habits must be particularly advised in psychosomatic disturbances of digestion.

There are two common energetic patterns of disharmony in the Earth functions that lead to gastralgia or stomach ulcers: deficiency of the Yin, and deficiency of the Yang aspect of the Spleen, respectively. The Metal Greater Yin type of pattern, in which the "child" of the Spleen, the Lung, is deficient, will entail deficient Yang of the Spleen, with aversion to cold, where body fluids and dampness (mucus) are not properly metabolized, often partly because of the overingestion of raw or cold food and cold drinks. In such cases the signs of deficiency of the Spleen Yang function will be accompanied by shooting abdominal pain, incessant diarrhea, and cold extremities, leading to a chronic, cold condition, often associated with colitis. The cold type of disorder serves as a predisposition to chronic stomach ulcers and stomach cancer, due again to deficiency of Yang of the Spleen.

The second common pattern is damp-heat, in which a deficiency of the Yin (Water, moisture) of the Spleen allows for an accumulation not only of mucus but also of heat, with gastric ulcers, dyspepsia, reflux esophagitis, and hiatus hernia (invasion by Liver-Gallbladder). Requena stresses the usefulness, in such cases, of the Spleen point that opens the Chung Mo Extra Meridian, namely Spleen 4, which is also the connecting point of the Spleen and carries Yin nourishing energy throughout the thorax by way of the Chung Mo network. This is associated with the front point for the Spleen and for Yin energy in general, namely Liver 13.[13]

In cases due to deficient Yang of the Spleen one must use "harmonizing" strategies, and heat points on the front and back for the Spleen function with moxibustion, burning an herb over or near points to increase Yang energy.

Just as the Earth-Metal Yin meridian system (Greater Yin, Lung and Spleen) often figures in gastric disturbances, its Yang-paired system, Sunlight Yang (Large Intestine and Stomach) will also often be involved. In such cases there will be an accumulation of improperly digested foodstuff in the Stomach, leading to heat and a feeling of energy rising up through the esophagus and throat to the head (through points Stomach 18, 12, 9, and 8). Western disorders showing this pattern are reflux esophagitis and heartburn. Persons suffering from this excess heat condition in the Stomach often complain of heartburn, which not infrequently turns out to be a heart attack taking the Xu Li (Stomach 18 to the Heart) pathway.

A passage in the *Yellow Emperor's Classic* gives specific symptoms for the various forms of Sunlight Yang digestive and intestinal complaints:

> When there is Yang heat in the Stomach the patient is always hungry and the skin above the navel is hot. In cases of heat in the Large Intestine, the skin below the navel is cold. In the case of Yin of the Stomach, the abdomen is swollen. In Yin of the Large Intestine, the patient has borborygmus or diarrhea and when there is Yin of the Stomach and Heat in the Large Intestine, there will be a swollen abdomen with diarrhea. When there is Yang of the Stomach and Yin of the Large Intestine the patient is always hungry and the lower abdomen is painful.[14]

Wood patterns, especially accompanied by anger or repressed rage causing constriction in the region controlled by the Liver in the pit of the Stomach (Conception Vessel 10 and 11, two or three inches directly above the navel), and known as "constrained Liver Qi," will often accompany Spleen deficient cases of gastralgia. In such Wood involvement, there will also be symptoms such as a bitter taste in the mouth and tightness or pain in the region of the rib cage and chest (controlled by Wood), perhaps involving gallstone formation. Perforated or seriously advanced acute ulcerous conditions frequently involve the Liver and Gallbladder Organ functions, with sharp stabbing pains in the pit of the stomach, spitting up of blood, sweating, and a congested feeling in the head as this heat escapes upward by way of the Stomach and Gallbladder channels. Modern Chinese medical research has shown extremely successful treatment of advanced, even perforated, ulcers with acupuncture alone, in sixty-five percent of the cases treated.[15]

While stomach disorders of the Sunlight Yang and Greater Yin types (involving Stomach, Spleen, and Large Intestine Organ functions primarily) often occur due to faulty eating habits such as rapid eating, eating standing up or at different times every day, or eating foods that are too cold, too greasy, or spicy, thus leading to "stomach distress," the specifically psychosomatic "nervous stomach" types of disorders will usually occur either from a primary excess and hyperactivity in Wood (Liver and Gallbladder functions), which invades and injures Spleen and Stomach functions, or from a deficiency of Yin of the Spleen, where the normally functioning Liver-Gallbladder system "overcontrols" and hence hinders the digestive Earth functions. In such cases, along with suggestions about diet and eating habits, it is essential to suggest calming activities like meditation, visualization, or biofeedback, which the patient can do independently whenever the constriction in the pit of the stomach begins (an "angry," as opposed to "distressed," stomach).

A powerful image I have found to be useful for people suffering from these sorts of digestive complaints, in which there is a constricted or pre-ulcerous condition in the stomach, is that of a constantly active, agitated, "angry" sympathetic system, ready at all moments for "fight or flight" because of fast-paced urban living and pressures. No fight or flight ensues, leading not to the normal parasympathetic reprieve in which the organism sinks into a deep resting phase to digest and take care of internal functioning but to an invasion of the parasympathetic system (Earth and Metal) by the sympathetic system, which is constantly being frustrated (Wood). This image is often sufficient, with only a handful of acupuncture treatments, to break the somatic compliance in the pit of the Stomach, and sometimes leads to recognition by the patient that he or she has been acting like a sympathetic type (the Type A person, in this case involving the Fire of Absolute Yin and Lesser Yang and Greater Yang functions, namely Pericardium, Triple Heater, and Small Intestine systems) when, in fact, the patient really longs for a parasympathetic (non–Type A) behavior and lifestyle. In such a case, the patient learns to recognize the constriction in the pit of the Stomach as the bodymind's way of requesting reprieve. He acknowledges that he neither cares for himself nor ever lets anyone else take care of him, and is subsequently better able to give up this "needy" stomach and look after himself. Truly restful vacations often prove of enormous value in such cases.

SECRET PLEASURES

From a psychosomatic perspective, anality is at the other end, liter-ally, of the oral–anal continuum occupying the first year and a half of life.

Anal eroticism is dealt with at length in the psychosomatic litera-ture and is summed up well by Alexander who shows that the infant early learns that "the other end of the intestinal tract can supply plea-sure similar to that which [the child] has known from suckling. This is caused by the pressure of a solid body on the mucous membrane of the anus and by the retention of the fecal mass."[16]

This explains the difficulty of toilet training, for the child is being asked to give up this secret pleasure.

An anal retentive reaction during the anal phase of psychosexual development will lead to stubbornness, independence, and posses-siveness, Alexander shows. In such cases the child "experiences plea-sure in withholding the products of his body to which no one but himself has access."[17] Feces are the child's first concrete, physical pos-session, and are only given up when rewards such as praise, sweets, or the like are offered by the mother. The relationship of anal eroti-cism to independence is key, as the issue of control of the anal sphinc-ter and other muscles arises when the child learns to hold and grasp objects. "He retains or surrenders at will," Alexander notes, "and resists or yields to adult pressure."[18] Severe interference with an in-fant's oral cravings is often compensated for by a later retentive atti-tude: "Since I didn't get what I wanted, and probably never will, I will hold on for dear life to what I have!"

The anal phase can be further broken down into retentiveness and elimination or expulsion. While anal retentiveness is associated with possessiveness and independence, the person shaped by a primary anal expulsive reaction pattern will have a kind of easily hurt pride and react with anal sadism, namely a desire to soil or defame. The anal and oral stages overlap imperceptibly, Alexander concedes, and it is merely the situation of toilet training that makes it appear as if the anal stage follows the oral stage. After weaning, toilet training is the second major interference with the child's normal bioenergetic functioning, whence its importance to psychosomatic analysis and treatment.

From a psychosomatic perspective, excremental functions are sec-ond only to ingestion of food as core functions around which somatic compliance may develop.

The key emotional constellation in orality is the desire for security, receiving, and taking by force what is not freely given, a desire to be loved and cared for, to lean on someone, to incorporate and be nourished by another.

The eliminative act, for its part, brings into play issues of possessiveness, pride in accomplishment, and giving versus retaining.[19] Hostile desires to attack and soil are often involved in this behavioral and personality predisposition. Alexander explains the psychosexual energetics thus: weaning → end of pleasurable sensations of sucking → thumb sucking as a replacement, which is thwarted by adults → discovery of pleasure in retention of a solid body (like sucking) → independence, which adults try to interfere with by toilet training → regularization → compliance with adult wishes in which excretion is seen unconsciously as a donation or gift to adults. The child first relates to excrement as a valuable possession, which is then transformed into its opposite, into something disgusting and dirty. Unconsciously, the act of defecation becomes sadistic and soiling in nature, as witnessed in the expression "Shit on you!"

LETTING GO

The common disorders cited in the psychosomatic literature that stem from conflicts in the anal stage are chronic diarrhea, spastic colon, and mucous colitis.

Chronic diarrhea is seen as a local pathological disturbance concomitant with psychic disturbance. Often it is presented by the patient as a central concern, the focus of constant worry and anxieties (worry and anxiety injure the Middle Zone in acupuncture energetics).

Mucous colitis is attributed to excessive parasympathetic activation (the Earth-Metal functions in acupuncture), with a personality configuration that includes overconscientiousness, dependence, hypersensitivity, anxiety, guilt, and resentment.

Alexander cites the presence of strong dependent wishes, and the urge to give, in most intestinal complaints studied by himself and his colleagues. These wishes substitute diarrhea for real accomplishment and giving. Often this takes the form of worrying about one's duties, obligations, and responsibilities; the need to provide money or support to others; the need to make an effort and do productive work, with a definite sense of overconscientiousness. In contrast to the peptic ulcer patient discussed earlier, who truly does exert himself, the diarrhea patient overcompensates for passivity through the unconscious association of the excremental act with giving.

Spastic colon and ulcerative colitis are different, Alexander maintains. In these disorders, marital discord is often a key precipitating factor, as are sexual conflicts and issues of pregnancy and abortion, financial obligations beyond one's means, and the general feeling of a need to accomplish something for which one is poorly prepared.

A key factor never to be forgotten in these intestinal complaints, Alexander adds, is the extent to which psychological rather than somatic factors are involved. The somatic functional disturbance cannot be ignored for the solely psychic dynamics, and, as we have already stated, acupuncture therapy is a precise and effective modality of treatment to break this somatic compliance.

Psychogenic constipation, another common disorder treated by the psychoanalysts of the 1930s, often occurs in people who betray a pessimistic, defeatist attitude; distrust and lack of confidence in others; and feelings of being unloved and rejected. This can go so far as to entail clinical paranoia or severe depression: ("I cannot expect anything from anyone, and therefore do not need to give anything. I must hold on to what I have!"). Alexander found that this condition succumbed very rapidly to short-term psychotherapy, whereas chronic diarrhea and colitis proved to be far more complicated and necessitated long-term analysis.

THE ACUPUNCTURE ENERGETICS OF ANALITY

The functions of the colon and elimination call to mind associations in Chinese medicine such as these: the Organ Functions of Metal, namely Lung and Large Intestines; grieving, loss, letting go or not being able to let go; and the Greater Yin and Sunlight Yang systems.

Intestinal complaints involving Wood are generally not serious (where fullness of Wood insults Metal against the normal control cycle). An example is fullness of the Gallbladder function with bouts of violent abdominal pains, alternating diarrhea and constipation, biliary vomiting, Gallbladder meridian headaches, hemorrhoids, or constipation, all due to heat in the Gallbladder system. These disorders clear up quickly with acupuncture therapy, combined with simple dietary restrictions to eliminate foods harmful to the Gallbladder.

Absolute Yin (Liver) Wood disturbances of intestinal function are similar to those involving the Gallbladder function—especially right-sided intestinal blockages with Liver invading the Spleen, leading to undigested food particles and loose stools, and alternating diarrhea and constipation. Requena states that treatment of Chung Mo, which traverses the intestinal region and strengthens the Spleen function, is often conclusive, with the addition of the points Spleen 4 (Chung Mo Thrusting Channel opening point) and Pericardium 6 (Yinweimo Yin Regulating Vessel opening point, as it is paired with Chung Mo and begins internally in the intestines).

In cases of Water involvement, frequently there will occur deficiency of Yang of the Kidney leading to bloody colitis and severe abscesses. Water-Fire (Kidney–Heart and Bladder–Small Intestine) disturbances resulting in intestinal complaints are far more serious. These include severe and chronic constipation and diarrhea, as well as Crohn's disease. In these cases either the Greater Yang or Lesser Yin meridian systems must be treated constitutionally. We have also seen that excessive sexual activity, often of the "false Fire" type, and excessive intake of cold drinks and foods (*especially ice cream*), are major contributing factors.

The most frequent disturbances noted in the acupuncture literature involving intestinal dysfunctions are fullness or weakness of the Large Intestine function itself.

In fullness there will be sharp pain on the left side, swelling, abdominal noises, constipation, and mucous or dry stools. In weakness or emptiness of the Large Intestine function, there will be an atonic colon, such as is found in older people or after debilitating surgery, or as a sequela to long-term fullness of this function, with very little actual pain, but slow motility. The Large Intestine will be more affected in the Fall and Winter because of cold, which leads to periumbilical pain and aversion to the cold.

Sunlight Yang forms of colitis (Stomach and Large Intestine functions) easily become chronic, usually occur on the left, and can easily lead to diverticulitis or fistulas. Nausea and loss of appetite will often occur as well, as Sunlight Yang is paired with Greater Yin (Spleen).

In Spleen disorders of intestinal functioning, there will be constipation in obese persons (with deficient Yin of the Spleen), and diarrhea due to deficient Yang of the Spleen, with watery, loose stools.

The key acupuncture point in this form of diarrhea is Stomach 25, two inches directly lateral to the navel on each side. Self-administered pressure or the application of a heating pad often proves very beneficial.

While disorders of gastrointestinal functioning are commonly and effectively treated by acupuncture, this is an area where the underlying psychodynamics are so evident as to warrant intervention by the acupuncture therapist on the side of the psyche directly.

A knowledge of the acupuncture energetics of the middle zone, coupled with an understanding of the various psychosomatic dynamics (the stress response, orality, dependence–independence issues) enables the bodymind-energetic acupuncture therapist to enter into a more integrated dialogue with the patient, aimed at discovering the significance of the distress in the digestive or intestinal functions. We have found that such an educational approach is often decisive, with changes occurring solely from the presentation of an integrated

acupuncture-energetic and psychosomatic explanation of the presenting complaint, as the following case will demonstrate.

ORGAN JET LAG

This metaphoric use of acupuncture-energetic imagery served as a
point of departure for this patient's recollection process.

A stewardess in her early thirties, whom I had seen on several previous occasions just before or after difficult flights to prevent the deleteri-
ous effects of jet lag, came to me for what she thought might be a
stomach virus. She appeared pale and exhausted when she entered
the office and had had no appetite, a frequent symptom of hers, for
days.

Palpation revealed extreme tightness and soreness all around the
navel and a very weak pulse in the positions associated with the Spleen
(Earth) and Kidney (Water) energetic functions. Her tongue was pale
with scallops around the edge, indicating a deficiency of Spleen energy.

She had been suffering for days from extreme bloating just below
the navel, chilliness throughout her body, and nausea.

I explained to her the energetics of the Spleen and its association
with the Earth Element in acupuncture theory. I also explained how
a deficiency of the Fire (Yang) of the Spleen often entails a deficiency
of the Fire (Yang) of the Kidneys. These two functions together move
food and fluids throughout the bodymind, preventing waterlogging
or accumulations of fluid or mucus. I discussed the other common
symptoms of a deficiency in these Yang functions of the Spleen and
Kidney, such as loose stools or diarrhea containing undigested food
particles (since the mother of the Spleen, namely, the Small Intestine's
Fire, cannot nourish the Spleen Fire function, leading to an inability
to break down and digest foods properly). She had been suffering
from these symptoms as well. I went on to discuss the more psychological aspects of the Small Intestine and Spleen Officials in acupuncture theory: the former related to the ability to prioritize things, to
establish clear values concerning what is of importance and what is
"crap" to be let go of; the latter related to the ability to focus, to be
centered, and to give and receive nourishment.

I finished by explaining that the main function of Spleen energy was
to hold organs in place, and that a common occurrence of Deficient
Spleen Energy could be seen in many women after giving birth, when
the heavy bleeding and exhausting labor lead to a significant deficiency
of Spleen Energy and Blood, with sinking internal organs such as a
dropped uterus, a dropped bladder, or anal prolapse.

She grew visibly excited at this point, exclaiming that many of her stewardess friends had shared a common complaint they termed "sagging insides." When they mentioned to their physicians that they felt empty in the middle, as if their insides had dropped down below the waist, they were met with marked skepticism and told they were just tired. Using this acupuncture imagery, she speculated about the way in which her career would necessarily weaken the Spleen's ability to hold up the insides, since she was obliged regularly to leave the Earth, thereby breaking the relationship between the Spleen and its primary Element. Not only were stewardesses obliged to lose touch with the Earth; while in flight, they were called upon to perform *the Earth function* for passengers, serving them food, reassuring them, *mothering* them! With a Spleen Official already weakened because of this separation from the Earth, a stewardess, nonetheless, is called upon to utilize what Spleen energy she has left, thereby depleting this energy further. Not only that, she added, but when the plane lands, everyone else is either back home or in some exotic land, while the stewardess is destined to spend a few hours in a hotel room trying to restore her energy for the return flight. Then she is obliged to leave Earth once again, and perform as the Spleen Official for another planeload of people before she can, at last, return to Earth and gain contact with her own center.

No wonder, my patient concluded, that stewardesses suffer from sagging internal organs and absorption problems. No wonder they often lose their appetites or, on the other hand, eat excessively, since their middle zone is totally off center.

She further felt that many stewardesses had ambivalent relationships with the Earth Element in the first place, which might explain in part their choice of profession. Their peripatetic lifestyle and search for the exotic could be seen as a denial of home, a refusal to be at ease in themselves.

In this instance I treated according to traditional acupuncture protocol with such points as the Fire and Earth points of the Spleen (Spleen 2 and 3), to tonify the Fire (Yang) of the Spleen and strengthen its functions, and the Fire and Earth points of the Kidney as well, to build the bodymind's internal Fire Root. This was coupled with Liver 13, a point under the rib cage, directly over the Liver and Spleen organs respectively, and Conception Vessel 12, over the Stomach, to direct the energetic effect of the treatment to the middle zone and prod the bodymind to function in this zone, and finally, Pericardium 6, on the Pericardium meridian, which connects with the meridian's internal pathway as it travels down the throat and esophagus to the Stomach and Intestines. By the time the needles were inserted, however, the treatment was already well under way, as the recollection and associations that occurred during the foregoing discussions are at the crux of gastric complaints such as hers. Acupuncture in such a case consolidates this recollection and situates its effects squarely within the body.

This woman continues to return for pre- or post-flight treatments, in order, as she now puts it, to be "grounded."

NOTES

1. W. B. Cannon, as quoted by Dunbar, *Emotions and Bodily Changes*, p. 272.
2. W. B. Cannon, as quoted in Dunbar, Ibid., p. 273.
3. Roy R. Grinker, *Psychosomatic Conflicts*. New York, Jason Aronson, 1973, p. 118.
4. Ibid., p. 119.
5. Ibid., pp. 119–122 for the above discussion.
6. Ibid., p. 124, quoted in Grinker.
7. Ibid., p. 126.
8. Ibid., p. 140.
9. Alexander, *Psychosomatic Medicine*, p. 48.
10. As quoted in Dunbar, Ibid., p. 284. Note that atonic constipation is due, in acupuncture, to a deficiency of Lung Energy in particular, and overall energy in general; Metal (Large Intestine and Lung functions) is the child of Earth (Stomach and Spleen functions).
11. Alexander, p. 104.
12. Ziegler, *Archetypal Medicine*, p. 104.
13. Cf. Requena, *Terrains et Pathologie*, for more details on the tai yin patterns.
14. As quoted by Requena, *Terrains et Pathologie*, our translation.
15. Journal of Chinese Medicine, Peking, No. 1, January 1974.
16. Franz Alexander, *Fundamentals of Psychoanalysis*, p. 50.
17. Ibid.
18. Ibid.
19. Alexander, *Psychosomatic Medicine*, p. 116.

9

Phenomenology of the Lower Zone: Genitourinary Functions

> . . . it is noteworthy that certain leading gynecologists, although fundamentally ignorant of or opposed to psychoanalysis, are nonetheless reaching the conclusion on the basis of their own observation and experience, that the majority of gynecological problems . . . are problems of psychosexuality.[1]
>
> Flanders Dunbar

Dunbar begins her chapter on the genitourinary and gynecological systems by remarking that the overlap between the two systems, at least in women, is so great as to warrant a unified investigation. The close relationship between micturition and sexuality—for example in the link between bedwetting and sexual anxiety dreams—was frequently noted by gynecologists and psychoanalysts of the early twentieth century.

In discussing the relationship between sterility and uterine fibroids, Kehrer, a leading German gynecologist of the 1920s, arrived at conclusions not dissimilar from those of classic psychosomatics and attributed gynecological dysfunctions to chronic disturbances in psychosexuality "with resulting chronic disturbances in abnormal blood and lymph distribution."[2] This view closely parallels the acupuncture-energetic explanation of gynecological and urinary complaints, which maintains that a disturbance in pelvic circulation of Blood or Energy may lead to accumulations known as stagnant Qi or congealed Blood, with accompanying lumps, cysts, or tumors.

The most important genitourinary organ-functional systems in Chinese medicine are the Liver, Spleen, and Kidney functions and meridians. Since the Liver is affected by anger or repressed rage, the Spleen by worry or anxious doubt, and the Kidney by fear, it is not surprising that genitourinary complaints involving these systems also entail psychic conflicts. Therefore, the experience of Western acupuncture therapists seems to corroborate that of the early psychosomatic analysts, in that emotions and the circulation of Blood and lymph fluids combine in the generation of all sorts of complaints converging on the lower, pelvic zone.

In 1927, Heyer, a prominent gynecologist, made the then radical statement that "a gynecologist who fails to see the effects of psychic factors in each situation is blind indeed."[3] Heyer went on to say that "[t]o a greater degree than any other physician the gynecologist is forced to be acquainted with the psychosomatic being of the woman instead of the pathological anatomy of the female genitalia. Departing from the usual cauterization, douching, and curetting which by focusing attention on the genitals only makes the condition worse, we must come more and more to see and treat in many gynecological disturbances the expression of psychic dysharmonies, especially of an erotic-sexual nature."[4]

A noted German gynecologist, Mayer, cites the work of Liepmann, Sellheim, and Kehrer, to the effect that "too much minor gynecology is being done and too little etiological thinking" and that "we treat the female organs much too much."[5] Dunbar herself concludes that "[many] of our patients present gynecological symptoms without being sick gynecologically. Their illness is a psychic conflict sailing under a gynecological flag . . ."[6]

We have repeatedly observed this to be true in the practice of acupuncture therapy as well, as the following case demonstrates.

A CASE OF PSYCHOSEXUAL URETHRITIS

A woman in her late 30s came for acupuncture treatment of what was variably diagnosed as cystitis or urethritis, after repeated courses of long-term antibiotic treatment were of no avail. She was extremely high-strung, and was disturbed by the recent loss of a high-paying, prestigious executive position, and her man friend's decision to break up their relationship of four years. She and her friend had decided to separate several times before, and each time they would subsequently engage in a frenzied period of passionate sexual activity, sex always having been the major attraction between them. The woman's pelvic symptoms—itching, irritation, low-grade fever, and achiness, often accompanied by a rise in her hypertensive condition and swelling of her breasts with tightness in the throat—would return promptly with each of these incidents. It was as if the rage at her friend, repressed during these passionate episodes, would concentrate its force on the psychosexual zone most threatened by his imminent departure.

Like acupuncture, classic psychosomatics essentially views disorders of the genitourinary functions as stemming from a damming up of energy in the pelvic zone, hindering proper circulation and elimination and leading to build-up and blockage of blood and fluids. Whether this dammed-up energy is due to repressed rage, resignation, regret, or indifference to the genitourinary functions involved, the result is an accumulation of noxious (stagnant, congealed) blood and lymph, rendering this lower zone a prime site for inflammation, irritation, and accumulations.

A combination of acupuncture therapy, to move the stagnant blood and energy, with appropriate, often short-term psychotherapy, seems of particular benefit in such disorders. Its efficacy was demonstrated in the case of a woman referred by her psychotherapist for concurrent acupuncture therapy, with multiple complaints including cystic breasts, premenstrual syndrome, migraines, mood swings, a knot in the pit of her stomach, periodic deep depressions, and a general sense of impending ill health. In the course of the acupuncture therapy, conducted once monthly for more than a year, many of her complaints were resolved or diminished in intensity and frequency. We shall explore this case in detail at the conclusion of this chapter to provide the reader with a sense of the potential for acupuncture therapy, practiced from a bodymind-integrative perspective, in a whole array of gynecological disturbances.

Given that the whole of the psychoanalytic perspective is based on a highly elaborated concept of psychosexual functioning, it is not surprising that the psychoanalytic literature on sexual disorders is so rich. The reader is referred to the work of Dunbar, and to that of Alexander and his colleagues, for a detailed discussion. We shall content ourselves in the following pages with a survey of the most common complaints and core issues involved.

THE TIP OF THE UTERUS

Referring to disturbances of menstruation in general, Dunbar notes "the far-reaching influence of psychic factors on the triad bleeding, pain, and leucorrhea,"[7] the most frequent complaints leading women to their gynecologists.

In the 1930s, it was frequently observed that psychotic patients showed a high degree of menstrual irregularities and, conversely, that irregular behavior could arise as a result of menstrual disorders, often referred to as "menstrual neuroses." Schindler reported on cases of "war amenorrheas" and believed that in many instances they were due not only to the stresses of wartime and lack of proper nourishment, but also to the unavailability of men. Frequently, he noted, regular menstruation would return as soon as men were present, even in the absence of sexual intercourse.[8]

The possibility of influencing the menstrual cycle by hypnotic suggestion was demonstrated consistently in the literature cited by Dunbar. Often one session was sufficient to regulate a cycle permanently. Hypnosis was sought regularly by women who feared that their period would come at an inopportune time, "as with girls intending to go to a ball, who often protect themselves with amulets . . . or with women who have one possible occasion for a long-desired intercourse."[9]

Acupuncturists in the West have often had similar experiences, with their female clients frequently asking for help in hastening or delaying the onset of a cycle for any number of social or personal reasons. As in the case of hypnosis, acupuncture therapy is very fast-acting in the regulation of the cycle, often requiring only a few sessions to achieve lasting results.

I am reminded of the case of an athlete in her early 20s who sought acupuncture treatment to help bring on her cycle, which had always been extremely erratic and had been absent for the past nine months. She wanted to become pregnant within the year, and her gynecologist, familiar with amenorrhea in athletes and dancers, suggested that she do less physical exercise and gain twenty pounds, shifting the hormonal balance in favor of a return of her cycles. Unable to do this without jeopardizing her career, she sought acupuncture therapy on the advice of a friend, and her period returned after one treatment. She continued to receive treatment once a week to ensure a normal second cycle, with two further treatments, a month apart, after that. Without changing her exercising or eating habits and without gaining any weight, this woman has now had regular cycles for the past eight months with only two return visits, on two different occasions, when she felt her period was a bit late. I have personally found acupuncture therapy to be so successful in restoring normal menstrual cycles where no irreversible organic cause is present, as well as in helping women become pregnant who had been unable to conceive for months or years, that I tell new patients coming for these complaints to be ready for a normal cycle to return within forty-eight hours, or pregnancy to take place within a few months, and I have not had to alter these "suggestions" for the past five years.

The positive suggestion itself works to enhance the power (or placebo *capacity*, depending on one's point of view) of the acupuncture treatment. In fact, it often leads women to develop visualization techniques of their own (the pelvis growing warmer, or a warm viscous fluid streaming through the pelvic region, or old dried-up blood being readied for expulsion), which, again, increase the effects of the therapy. I have also observed traditionally trained Oriental practitioners treat women with the same complaints, using no suggestion and not so much as a word of explanation about the energetics involved in the disrupted cycles, with consistently good results. The mere placement of needles along the energetic pathways (Spleen, Kidney, and Liver channels, primarily) that traverse and energize the pelvic zone appears to be sufficient for stimulating more normalized energetic (and hence hormonal) functioning. Nevertheless, suggestion and visualization techniques, as well as the appropriate counseling, are in order, for these bodymind methods help prevent further disturbances of this energetic zone in the future and enable patients to regain control of their own bodies.

A point of clarification is in order lest the reader begin to suspect that I am agreeing with an obviously male chauvinistic psychoanalytic perspective that tends to see women's illnesses, far more often than men's, as psychological in origin. It must be emphasized that the authors just cited were in many cases gynecologists hostile to the psychoanalytic perspective, who nonetheless were unable to deny the close link between psyche and soma in gynecological complaints. Male genitourinary complaints appeared far less frequently in the literature, as we shall discuss somewhat later, but at this point it is important to reflect on the evidently greater frequency in women than in men of a clearly overt relationship between the mind and the bodily functions in genitourinary complaints such as those given here.

First, the reader will be reminded that one thesis of the bodymind-energetic approach is that a combined use of psychosomatic and acupuncture-energetic perspectives may be justified precisely because both start from the premise, which is consistently found to be true in practice, that the mind and body are always inextricably linked in any physical complaint, no matter how minor. There is no separation between the psyche and the body, and when we speak of a disorder's psychological aspects, this can never be construed as a denigration of the patient. While it is true that many medical practitioners today use the word "psychosomatic" far more frequently with women than with men (to mean that their patients are "crocks" or their disorders "imaginary" and "only in their heads"), this is due to a deplorable ignorance on the part of the medical community of the nature of, and links between, psyche and soma—links the early psychosomatic physicians were trying to elucidate. That these early physicians were also psychoanalysts, and therefore influenced by Freudian psychosexual theories that are falling ever more into disrepute in our day, obviously colored their work and led to overly psychosexual interpretations. The bodymind-energetic approach avoids this aspect of the classic psychosomatic perspective because of the sexual biases inherent in it. This does not mean that one must ignore the psychosomatic literature itself.

Second, it should not surprise us that women would have more overt bodymind disorders of the lower zone, for the simple reason that the menstrual period itself is so easily construed as an "evil" or "sickness" in traditional as well as modern societies. Bleeding tends to be associated with illness, and hence in a young girl it is likely that her initial reaction to this new process is psychologically complicated. She may wonder what this bleeding is all about; whether she will be found more attractive, or on the contrary repellent; whether she can still engage in all of the same physical activity; and what this new capacity to become pregnant means to her. These are some of the questions that a young girl may ask herself at the start of her menses. The questions and concerns are psychological as well as physical in and of themselves, and sufficient to bring about pelvic disruptions. I have treated numerous college students who were sexually active yet practiced no form of birth control. When I expressed concern, they retorted that sex was not really a passionate activity for them, and that they never really "gave in" to their partners—either because sex didn't interest them that much or because they would not "give in" until they met the right man. In several of these cases the women became pregnant as soon as they had sex with men they were in love with. This demonstrated to me, early in my acupuncture work, that the mind can control the body.

Finally, it may be possible that modern women, for many sociocultural and perhaps even biological reasons, have developed somatic manifestations of psychic conflicts more readily than men because it is to their benefit. While men in many Western cultures have been trained to remain silent about the emotional and psychological conflicts they feel, thereby forcing these psychological energies deep into the body, women have often been afforded more space (often, unfortunately, in their doctor's office) for speaking out about their emotional and psychological stress. If a woman develops a splitting migraine at the onset of her period, with violent cramps and clotting and becomes ill-tempered, uninterested in sex with her husband, and perhaps even abusive toward him, it is possible that some aspects of these physical symptoms derive from an incredible rage toward him for being a man, for being the one who can leave and have a career while she is forced to stay at home and take care of the children and the household affairs. But migraines and cramps and mood-swings are rather benign physical symptoms in and of themselves, and perhaps serve as a regular way to let off steam, thereby preventing the frustration and anger from generating a more serious physical complaint. Her husband may well be feeling similar frustrations and anger at their relationship and at the need to go out and work, but in our culture it is still far more likely that he will refuse to express these psychological conflicts openly, thus driving them deep into his body and increasing the chance of developing explosive and potentially fatal physical disorders such as high blood pressure or a heart attack.

The point in all of these situations is that we all suffer from splits between mind and body, because we have been raised from childhood in a society that culturally and medically divides the two realms. As more and more medical and mental health practitioners develop a bodymind-integrative orientation, it will become essential to discuss openly and in great detail the psychological as well as physical aspects of clients' complaints. Incidentally, it may well be that those most readily (and derogatorily) diagnosed by their physicians as suffering from purely psychosomatic complaints will be the very people most capable of utilizing such mental means as relaxation, self-hypnosis, and imaging techniques to bring their physical symptoms under control.

This would already appear to be the case in what Dr. Bernie Siegel, a prominent surgeon who practices from a bodymind integrative perspective, terms the "exceptional cancer patient." These patients always accept the fact that their cancerous tumors developed on the basis of psychological as well as physical imbalances, and they sometimes are capable of making changes in both arenas to bring their cancers under control. Imaging techniques, which are a clear use of the mind to control the body, are among the most successful therapies in such patients. But no one would say that these patients are easy to get along with, for the simple reason, as Siegel points out, that they refuse to be traditional passive patients, demanding instead that the doctor or therapist carry out their desires as they choose: "Exceptional patients refuse to be victims. They educate themselves and become specialists in their own care. . . . Physicians must realize that the patients they consider difficult or uncooperative are those who are most likely to get well" owing, in large measure, to a "fighting spirit" rather than a "stoic acceptance" of their disease.[10]

With these comments in mind I should like to conclude this discussion of psychosomatic disorders of the pelvic zone with a look at two complicated problems, uterine fibroid tumors and *grossesse nerveuse*.

Frigidity and associated disorders of sterility and fibroid tumors were reported to be psychogenic by many psychosomatically inclined gynecologists of the early twentieth century, among them Kehrer and Mohr, prominent German gynecologists of that period.[11]

Kehrer maintained that fibroid formation does not lead to sterility, but rather that both are "coordinate sequelae of the same fundamental condition, i.e., chronically disturbed psychosexuality, with resulting chronic disturbances in abdominal blood and lymph distribution."[12] He found that fibroids developed most frequently in women with unsatisfactory sexual lives and that the bigger the fibroid, the earlier one could date the beginning of this dissatisfaction. Wengrof, a specialist in psychosomatic medicine at the turn of the century, noted that "a conflict coming from the genital" could lead to change in the tissues with a hypertrophy that later develops into a fibroma. In such conditions, he found that a brief course of psychotherapy was sufficient at times to retard or shrink the growth of the fibroids.[13]

Psychogenic, false pregnancy, or *grossesse nerveuse*, in which a woman maintains the outward signs of a pregnancy that does not exist and that may culminate in a mimicked labor, is a phenomenon observed and treated frequently by psychosomatic analysts and physicians.

A milder version of the same phenomenon takes the form of excessive bloating during menstruation, often associated with secret pregnancy fantasies, and has proved especially amenable to analytic treatment.

Dunbar concludes her own survey of gynecological disorders by quoting Mayer, a noted gynecologist, who underscored the responsibility of physicians treating women's complaints. First, Mayer pointed out, the physician "must remember that his every utterance and act, as well as every therapeutic measure, has a suggestive effect upon the patient, only too often of a harmful nature." He goes on to offer several examples of such negative suggestions: "a slight or unconsidered remark, e.g., about 'weak lungs' may give rise to a lasting fear of pregnancy, and thus result in frigidity and marital disharmony. The consciousness of a gynecological disease means to many women the reproach of sexual inadequacy with all its sequelae." He concludes, "Especially pernicious are the words 'inflammation of the ovary' and 'tip of the uterus.' 'Tip' to a great number of women connotes innumerable diseases, the certainty of serious disease, or working incapacity."[14]

Mayer's conclusions in 1925 hold true for today's gynecologists. "[T]here are all too many women carrying on their bodies numerous marks of treatment by specialists, *who still keep their complaints after being told again and again that anatomically everything was normal.* Whole series of procedures, such as operations, curettage, discission of the cervix, amputation of the portio, plastic operations, excision of the adnexae, appendectomies, nephropexies, gastroenterostomies, and finally extirpation of the uterus—all had been done in vain."[15] Anyone who thinks about this comes to the rapid conclusion that such procedures cannot eliminate the real source of the complaints. Mayer's comments will ring especially true to the many thousands of women today who have undergone hysterectomies performed too hastily, or without any counseling as to the often dramatic changes that may occur. When a physician cannot help someone, Mayer adds, this is unfortunate, "but when a woman who was previously gynecologically healthy becomes sick as a result of sequelae of an unnecessary operation, or even becomes incapacitated, or dies, we have the saddest results of a one-sided specialist's orientation, with failure to recognize psychogenic etiology of disease."[16]

Such a lack of recognition leads to overuse of gynecological procedures, even the simplest of which, such as frequent or lengthy local manipulations, may prove injurious. For such manipulations focus the attention of the patient on the physical complaint, unconsciously encouraging the patient to develop a real disorder. Witness the anxiety often experienced by women whose Pap smears show up positive and whose gynecologists, stressing the necessity of a Pap test in three or six months, say, inadvertently, "You wouldn't want us to miss anything, would you?" This admonition includes the suggestion "you will develop *something*." Unfortunately, Mayer's suggestions to the gynecologists and internists of his day went essentially unheeded, and his closing remarks are especially apropos today: "[i]f a new generation in medicine continues to consider every gynecological symptom as a sign of local disease, and a reason for local treatment, they will remain blind organ specialists staring at the uterus through a magnifying glass, overlooking the rest of the patient."[17]

Given the clear male chauvinism prevalent at the end of the nineteenth and beginning of the twentieth centuries in Europe and the United States, it is not surprising that the classic psychosomatic literature essentially discusses only female genitourinary complaints. Because of this, many men still refrain from admitting to dysfunctions in the pelvic zone, and doctors tend not to question their male patients as carefully as women concerning pelvic symptoms in a routine physical examination.

While it appears true that women do seek medical care more frequently than men for genitourinary complaints, the rise of a relatively new complaint—nonspecific prostatitis—in young men, not necessarily related to the more serious prostate disorders of older men, is not dissimilar to the vague and bothersome complaints that so frequently send some women to their doctors. Perhaps the sexual issues raised over the past two decades concerning male sexual oppression have been internalized by subsequent groups of young men, predisposing the male sexual organs to distress or disease. There is also a rise of vague and strange pelvic abnormalities such as swollen glands or nodules or rashes in men suffering what I have come to refer to as "fear of AIDS syndrome." These men, not necessarily gay, always have at least one friend who has been diagnosed with AIDS, or has succumbed to the disease, immediately before the onset of their own symptoms.

It is clear, therefore, that male pelvic distress and disease will come under greater scrutiny in the years to come, and a bodymind perspective, focused on the psychological as well as the somatic energetics involved, will be warranted.

I have often discovered genitourinary dysfunctions—such as mild forms of impotence, premature ejaculation, dribbling or frequent urination, and achiness or pain in the pelvic zone—in my male patients, who never thought of these imbalances as complaints to be brought to their physicians. In most cases these are not the complaints with which they come to me, but once they realize that they are symptoms of a more generalized energetic imbalance—say, of deficiency of Kidney Fire or Liver energy—they become willing to discuss their meaning. Psychosexual conflicts, such as loss of a female companion, fear of sexual inadequacy, guilt over having an extramarital affair, and so forth, often emerge in our discussions together. Such vague symptomatology often clears up very rapidly in acupuncture therapy, thereby preventing actual organic disorders later on.

ACUPUNCTURE PELVIC PATHWAYS

While acupuncture-energetic analysis clearly recognizes the crucial role of "maldistribution of blood and lymph" noted by Kehrer, it is essentially inarticulate concerning the psychosexual factors involved, undoubtedly because of the "puritanism" of the Chinese approach to sexuality in general. However, the acupuncture-energetic perspective does provide a clear and detailed description of the energetic relationships between the three organ-functions whose respective meridians traverse and energize the pelvic zone: the Spleen, Liver, and Kidney functions.

The Spleen Official is considered to be affected by worry and doubt, the Liver Official by anger or repressed rage, and the Kidney Official by fear and problems with authority. Thus it can be seen that the acupuncture perspective takes into account the same emotional conflicts as classic psychosomatics.

What follows is a summary of the major acupuncture-energetic patterns of dysfunction of the lower zone.

ENERGETIC DISTURBANCES OF
THE LOWER ZONE

The Three Yin channels of the Foot all converge, a few inches above the internal ankle bone, at the point Spleen 6 (called "Three Yin Crossing"), and again just above the pubic bone, at Conception Vessel 2 and 3. Here these meridians plunge deep into the pelvic zone. The Liver channel skirts the external genitalia, and all three channels traverse the uterus and ovaries, or the prostate, bladder, and kidneys, before surfacing to flow up through the breast region.

Therefore, genitourinary disorders in Chinese medicine are attributed to some combination of disturbances in these three functions, with a concomitant disturbance in vital substances in the pelvic zone (deficiency, stagnation, accumulation, or heat affecting the Blood, Qi, or Fluids).

In dysmenorrhea, for example, three common patterns are frequently discerned in the Oriental medical literature. First, painful menstruation is attributed to stagnant Energy and congealed Blood, where a deficiency of Energy in general (related to deficiency of the Lung Qi) leads to poor circulation of Blood and results in accumulation of "congealed Blood" in the pelvic region (the Lung is the "child" of the Spleen; hence, deficiency in Energy, under control of the Lungs, will drain the "mother," the Spleen). If only Qi is stagnant, such accumulations may include soft movable cysts, whereas in the case of congealed blood hard immovable masses such as fibroids or tumors may be present. Signs of such pelvic complaints may include a swollen, painful abdomen; irregular menstrual flow; dark flow with clots; relief from the pain after passing the clots; swollen breasts; a purple tongue; and a wiry pulse. The pulse denotes a disturbance of the Liver channel, and in fact this energetic pattern is frequently combined with "Constrained Liver Qi" (sometimes due to a deficiency of Lung Qi, as noted above, in which the Lung Phase is too weak to control the Liver Phase properly). Often this is accompanied by anger, repressed rage, or other violent emotions that "hinder the smooth flow of Qi," under the control of the Liver Official. When the emotions are not on an even keel, as we saw in Chapter 2, the uterus, pelvic region, and genitals, all energized by the Liver channel, are prone to disturbances.[18]

Another common energetic pattern leading to dysmenorrhea is known as "Cold Damp Obstructing" the menstrual cycle because of a deficiency of the Yang function of the Spleen in transforming fluids and combating "dampness" and cold in the pelvic zone. In such cases the abdomen will be painful and cold to the touch. It may even feel "internally" cold, and the application of heat will help. The menses will be uneven, dark, and watery with some clots. The tongue will be pale (Deficient Spleen) and the pulse, sinking (Deficiency) or slow (Cold).

Finally, in the case of dysmenorrhea with Deficient Blood and Qi, circulation in the pelvic zone will be impaired with soreness in the abdominal region, which can be relieved by pressure. There will be a pale complexion; pale tongue; fatigue; scanty, pale blood; and a weak, thin pulse. Such a condition may be due to chronic fatigue or may occur after surgery or childbirth, or in a person besieged by emotional conflict involving obsessive worry or grief (injuring Earth or Metal, and hence Greater Yin functions of the Spleen and Lung).

These three patterns occur in many other pelvic complaints. For example, stagnant Qi and congealed Blood may also be at the root of amenorrhea, in which emotional stress and sudden cessation of menstruation occur, or of functional uterine bleeding, with chronic scanty bleeding or sudden heavy bleeding and other constrained Liver Qi signs like distended flanks and a wiry pulse, or of pelvic inflammatory disease also related to constrained Liver Qi.

Cold-Damp may be at the root of amenorrhea, in which mucus build-up, due to the deficiency of the Spleen's transforming functions, blocks the flow, resulting in weakness in the abdomen and other deficient Spleen signs like nausea, loss of taste or appetite and a slippery pulse. When this dampness (mucus) turns hot (leading to inflammation, a common result of damp obstructions), dribbling urination, urinary tract infections, pelvic inflammatory disease, and prostatitis may occur, with additional symptoms such as cloudy urine, distended abdomen, achiness in the pelvic zone, and a slippery pulse.

Deficient Blood and Qi are often involved in amenorrhea, in which the menstrual flow will gradually diminish and then stop, and in abnormal uterine bleeding, in which the deficient Spleen function cannot maintain the blood in the vessels, with weak legs and edema. Deficient Spleen and Kidney Yang functions often occur together and may lead to pelvic inflammatory disease with sore back, distended abdomen (where pain increases after exertion or sexual activity), and swelling of the lower extremities (deficient Yang of the Spleen function) and an aversion to cold (deficient Yang of the Kidney function).

Another pattern, which usually occurs as a result of a deficiency of Yin of the Kidney and Liver Organ functions, is heat in the blood, with a rapid pulse, red tongue, dark red heavy bleeding and urethritis. This occurs in some cases of amenorrhea, with a withering away of the person, dry scalp and skin, weak lower back and legs, and thirst. It occurs in abnormal uterine bleeding, and also in advanced or acute stages of pelvic inflammatory disease and urinary tract infections, with painful, urgent urination, warm palms and soles, and a dry mouth.

Urinary disorders such as dribbling (whether or not associated with prostatitis, pelvic inflammatory disease, or urinary tract infections) also may be due to the specific weakness of the Yang aspect of the Kidneys (the "life gate fire"), which is intimately connected with the Bladder functions and is fed by energy from the Yang of the Spleen. The Yang aspect is damaged, as in the case of Spleen Yang, by excessive worry, overexertion, mental or physical fatigue, or poor dietary habits. This deficiency of the Middle and Lower Zones often occurs in people who are physically active in their 20s but become sedentary in their 30s. This injures the ability of the Spleen Yang to absorb nutrients, thereby weakening the Center (governed by the Spleen Official). The organs in this region will then become weak, and even drop (the ptosis of various organs or hemorrhoids). Many patients suffering from these weaknesses report a feeling of emptiness in the center, or a feeling of cold, or as if everything were hanging down, often accompanied by flabbiness in precisely this zone. This deficiency can be corrected to a large extent by rest and more sleep, moderation of sexual and eating habits, abstention from alcohol, appropriate mild, toning exercises, and meditation to calm the mind.

From this summary we can see that an acupuncture-energetic perspective is rich in somatic-energetic explanations of genitourinary complaints, and can lead to highly specific and individualized treatment focusing on the precise zone (Liver, Spleen, Kidney) affected. Acupuncture treatment of these genitourinary disorders is very effective and is often conclusive in resolving these complaints. But in some instances, especially those involving symptoms of a chronic nature, short-term counseling or psychotherapy combined with the acupuncture therapy will yield the best results.

We shall conclude this survey of the lower zone with a bodymind-energetic analysis of a complex case involving the woman suffering from several functional gynecological complaints referred to early in this chapter.

A CASE OF WANDERING LIVER QI

A woman was referred to me by her psychotherapist for a multiplicity of physical complaints that had grown worse during her psychotherapy, and that he felt needed direct attention. She had self-diagnosed "premenstrual syndrome," with exquisitely painful breasts at ovulation and menstruation, severe menstrual cramps with heavy clotting, extremely strong sexual desires before her periods that she feared would engulf her if she gave in to them, and frequent migraines, especially at ovulation and before the start of her period.

She was very much aware of the variations in her symptoms with phases of her cycle, and joked in an early session that she must be mad since she was so influenced by lunar energies.

She often suffered from nausea, vague digestive complaints, and constipation. Her moods were variable, with occasional but severe bouts of "deep, sinking depression." Her bodily aches and pains were also variable, coming and going suddenly and traveling throughout her body, traversing at times the inner sides of the legs and thighs to the pelvic region, and at other times the outside of her legs and hips and sometimes attacking the pit of her stomach or middle back, as well as her head (migraines).

She seemed very concerned with her bodily symptoms, but was equally capable of making psychological associations or discussing the meaning of these symptoms.

When I discussed the notion of body/mind split with her, she admitted being closer to the side of the psyche and feeling more or less afraid of her actual physical forces and appetites. She related to her sexuality as a dark, mysterious, and ultimately deadly force, which she felt she always needed to keep under control. Her husband had very mild sexual desires, which helped her restrain her own passions. She was also very athletic and worked out at the gymnasium or jogged every day. Her body was lean and very muscular for the most part, but she had voluptuous breasts, which bothered her.

She thought of herself as quite intelligent and potentially very creative as a writer, but not especially good looking. (She was, in fact, strikingly attractive.)

In our discussions a litany of complaints would ensue that pointed to a real dislike of the body in general. This coincided with an almost ascetic relationship to eating and sleeping. In adolescence this patient had been diagnosed as mildly anorectic, but she showed little interest in discussing this stage in her health.

When I asked her to describe her menstrual pains, she reported that they were similar to an orgasm, deep and penetrating. Her periods would cease for months at a time, as had been the case from the onset of menstruation.

Palpation revealed a very wiry, taut pulse in the middle positions, related to Liver, Gallbladder, and Stomach functions, and a slightly deficient Spleen function pulse. The Liver meridian was tight, especially on the internal aspect of her lower legs, and along the midline, from just above the navel, through the ribcage and up to the throat. She was also very tight along the entire Gallbladder pathway, from the temples to the sides and back of her head and neck, to her sides, pelvic region, hips, and lateral aspect of the legs and ankles. She rarely perspired, even with excessive physical activity, which indicated a deficiency of the Triple Heater function, paired with the Pericardium and of the same nature as its lower, Gallbladder energetic unit (both Lesser Yang). She added in the initial interview that "everything" was wrong with her body, and that she also thought she might have a "tipped uterus."

The initial evaluation revealed an imbalance between Wood and Fire, bringing into play the Yin as well as the Yang functions, namely Lesser Yang (Gallbladder and Triple Heater) and Absolute Yin (Liver and Pericardium). She showed an almost total absence of anger at all times, with a greenish tinge to the face (Wood) and a lack of red in the complexion (deficient Fire). It appeared as if her Wood (Liver, Gallbladder) energy could not properly move to its child, the Fire Element (Pericardium, Triple Heater), because of constriction of this energy in the pelvic, digestive, and throat regions, which would indicate a diagnosis of "constrained Liver Qi" in modern Chinese medical terminology. The latter diagnosis would also account for her somewhat weak Spleen pulse, frequent nausea, loss of appetite, and bloating during her cycle—all symptoms of invasion of the Earth (Spleen) by an overactive or constricted Wood phase (Liver, in this case).

The somatic energetic-reactive zone most disturbed was clearly that of Lesser Yang (Gallbladder and Triple Heater), with muscular rigidity and armoring along its entire length and most of the symptoms

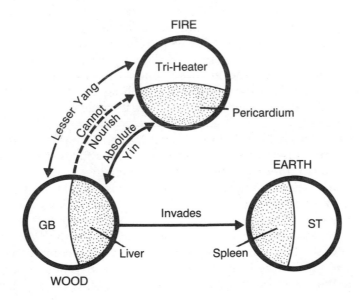

centering in this zone. Therefore I decided to commence treatment by opening this Lesser Yang zone to restore a more normal flow of energy deeper in her body. I explained these energetics to her, and suggested that once the energy from the surface, Lesser Yang zone was freed up, it would flow into its paired, deeper Yin zones (Liver and Pericardium, Absolute Yin).

In the first few treatments, spaced a week apart, she reacted intensely to the needling, feeling jolts of electricity streaming throughout her body, "not unlike an orgasm." Her reactions to the treatments always proved very strong, often with an exacerbation of symptoms along the Gallbladder or Triple Heater pathways (such as increased tension in the temples or occipital region, sudden intense headaches that would come and go, or sciatic pains). Within a few sessions she noticed that she was starting to perspire more easily (indicating that the Triple Heater function was being strengthened). After a month or so of weekly treatments, we scheduled treatments at one-month intervals to insure regular periods, prevent exaggerated symptoms during menstruation, and slowly begin to regulate this complex energetic field.

Within a few months her periods were regular and far less painful, and the swelling in her breasts decreased markedly. She was much less tense in general, with fewer dramatic reactions both at the time of treatment and in the period between treatments. She seemed to grow more fond of her body, and her general appearance became milder as the hard edge of the Lesser Yang reaction pattern was softened. Her migraines continued to decrease in frequency and severity, and her violent wandering pains were now more like mild aches or generalized sensations of constriction, which she could sometimes lessen with simple breathing or relaxation exercises we devised on the basis of imagery she discovered during her acupuncture sessions. The imagery usually aimed at allowing her pelvic and stomach constrictions to relax, and involved sending mild currents of purple and golden light from the pelvis to the diaphragm and chest, culminating in the throat and temple regions where it would course back down through the body.

She reported that her therapist was delighted with the progress she was making in her work, with discussions now focused on core dynamic issues rather than her physical complaints.

Once the Lesser Yang reaction pattern was sufficiently relaxed, I started to focus on the deeper, Absolute Yin functions, beginning primarily with the Liver and the "constrained Liver Qi." This yielded quickly to acupuncture treatment, at which point the Pericardium (Master of the Heart, or Heart Protector Official) function, of sending energy to protect the heart organ and ward off psychological stress, became the center of attention. Treatment of points such as Bladder

14, and the special point for spiritual disturbances of the Heart Protector function, according to some teachings, on the second line of the Bladder meridian lateral to Bladder 14, Pericardium 5 and 6, and Kidney 2 (to build the Fire Root of the Kidneys as well as the Heart Fire) proved very calming and bracing to her. During these treatments she would soften emotionally and speak of relationships, love, and her constant fear that sexual energy, if unleashed, would consume her in some dangerous fashion. This has become the focus of her work with her psychotherapist; at the time of this writing she is treated almost monthly, with continued improvement of her major symptoms as well as in her general approach toward life. She has turned her energy more seriously toward writing, and seems optimistic about her creative endeavors in particular and about the future in general, which used to fill her with fear.

NOTES

1. Dunbar, *Emotions and Bodily Changes*, p. 318.
2. As quoted in Dunbar, p. 342.
3. G. R. Heyer, as quoted in Dunbar, p. 332.
4. Ibid.
5. Ibid., as quoted in Dunbar, p. 332.
6. Ibid.
7. Ibid., p. 333.
8. Ibid.
9. Ibid., p. 334.
10. Bernie S. Siegel, *Love, Medicine and Miracles*, pp. 24–25.
11. Ibid., p. 339.
12. Ibid., p. 342.
13. Ibid.
14. As quoted in Dunbar, p. 349.
15. Ibid., p. 350 (emphasis ours).
16. Ibid.
17. Ibid., pp. 350–351.
18. For this, and all further discussion of patterns here, cf. Kaptchuk, *The Web That Has No Weaver*, pp. 296–299 and 329–333.

10

Phenomenology of
Musculoskeletal Reaction Patterns

In the little child the most primitive expression of frustration is random motor discharge.[1]

Alexander and French

The literature on the psychosomatics of the musculo-skeletal system,
especially low back syndrome and various forms of arthritis (specifically rheumatiod arthritis) is quite inconclusive.

Here, more than anywhere else, the weakness of the psychoanalytically inspired psychosomatic approach is evident, owing to the lack
of a somatic-energetic understanding and therapeutic methods that
would enable one to explain and treat the organ or site of somatization in such disorders.

MOTOR DISCHARGES

Alexander observes that "[i]n the little child the most primitive expression of frustration is random motor discharge. If, through primitive measures, this discharge becomes associated with fear and guilt,
in later life whenever fear and guilt arise there results a psychologic
straight jacket."[2]

In low back pain, such muscular discharge has been observed. In a case of psychogenic back pain reported by Saul,[3] a male patient with severe lumbar pain reported violent dreams of running, pounding, attacking, playing sports, and carrying heavy loads on his back—all associated with some "test" of his person involving heavy muscular activity. He would wake up with a rigid, tight back and crossed legs that were equally rigid and contracted. Whether these contractions caused the back pain or exaggerated an already weak back condition, Saul states, there might not have been any psychological meaning behind the pain; it might merely have been a correlative of the emotional tensions involved. Thus, when this man became tense and slept badly, his back would go into spasm.

Saul's explanation skirts the issue of why such tension couldn't as easily affect the neck instead, and he admits that a somatic weakness would have to be assumed. On the other hand, he continues, it is possible that there may be specific psychological factors involved in the selection of the back as the site for absorption of the tension. He cites Fetterman, who thought that this localization had to do with "the upright posture, implying adulthood with all its responsibilities and exertions."[4] Finally, Saul observes, there is an indication of sexual tension involved, in which pelvic congestion related to sexual tension can refer to the back. This can be seen also, for example, in the physiology of low back pain in women during menstruation.

In the case of rheumatoid arthritis, behavioral attempts to delineate a rheumatoid personality configuration have proved inconclusive as well. While it was found that women (who represent more than sixty-five percent of those suffering from the disease) appeared to be tense, moody, and unable to express anger, with "rejecting" mothers and "strict" fathers,[5] colitis patients shared the same factors. An interesting observation made by behaviorists is that since rheumatoid arthritis is an autoimmune disorder, "researchers have wondered whether a particular form of self-destructive personality might not translate into an autoimmune, neurophysiological self-destructiveness."[6] According to Pelletier, however, research is still far too sketchy to arrive at any specific conclusions in this regard.

The psychoanalytic literature on rheumatoid arthritis focuses primarily on the spastic state of the muscles in such conditions, related to a supposedly "chronic, inhibited, hostile aggressive state."[7]

While some investigators reported the arthritis to symbolize a punishment or atonement for "aggressive competitive feelings toward men,"[8] most psychoanalytic research seems to point, as did Groddeck's initial findings, to a "defense against the heterosexual role." This may easily be interpreted as an unconscious refusal to perform in society as a subjugated woman, this refusal affecting the very ability of the bodymind to move and behave in such a subjugated fashion.

The personality factors gleaned from the psychoanalytic literature point to "tomboyish behavior" in latency, with "strong control of all emotional expressions in adulthood."[9]

The women suffering from rheumatoid arthritis cited by Shapiro, Johnson, and Alexander showed a strong "masculine protest reaction" involving the adoption of "masculine competitiveness," a "competitive relationship with men." While the literature revealed any number of precipitating factors, a few specific psychodynamic factors were consistently present. Alexander noted that the arthritis developed during an increase in unconscious rebellion and resentment directed at men and was usually related to events that might tend to increase hostility and guilt feelings previously latent and adequately handled through the patient's self-sacrifice and service to others.[10] It is likely that what these early psychosomaticians called "masculine protest" was more specifically a feminist protest against inequality based on biological makeup.

In thirty-three cases, Alexander and his colleagues were able to note two dynamic situational patterns: rejection of the female function (the masculine protest reaction) often associated with manifest bisexuality, and a "masochistic need to do for others,"[11] which Alexander attributes to a discharge of this "protest" and a denial of the dependency on taking care of men and children in our culture.

The families of these women usually contained one strict or domineering parent and one subservient one, and these women started at an early age to place severe restrictions on themselves. Atonement for resentment against the mother, or rejection of her, was also frequently observed.

Alexander concludes that, strictly speaking, rheumatoid arthritis therefore falls into the category of hysterical conversion reactions, as an "expression of an unconscious conflict by somatic changes in the voluntary muscles."[12]

Alexander hypothesized that the muscle spasms, and resultant increased muscle tonus, predisposed the bodymind to arthritis attack.

Only in a few cases were Alexander and his coworkers able to observe specific unconscious tension within target organ systems that would account for the predisposition of these systems to spasm and ensuing arthritis.

The "psychological straight jacket" developed by these patients occurs as an attempt to create a balance between aggressive drives and a wish to control others. When different specific events come to interrupt the adaptive reaction patterns of these patients, thereby interrupting the discharge of hostility and relief from guilt, the muscle tonus increases and an arthritis attack is imminent.

While Alexander maintained that somatic (traumatic, infectious, or genetic) factors probably were involved in the predisposition toward arthritic attack in a precise location of the body, he added that there must be a combination of psychological conflictual situations as well as increased muscle tonus to initiate an attack.

Adopting a phenomenological perspective, Ziegler observed a specific phenomenological pattern in both men and women suffering from rheumatoid arthritis: a conflict between flexibility and "stoic immobility." He noted that these patients were perpetually active (always on behalf of others), self-effacing, extremely conscientious, and almost stoic. In analyzing the etymology of the words in German related to rheumatoid arthritis, Ziegler postulates that "all rheumatic loss of articulation could, in actuality, signify an increase in constancy and steadfastness. It is as if Nature were attempting to prevent an all-too-ready marionette-like adaptation, a tendency toward a jack-in-the-box identity."[13] While they may react externally in a submissive, self-effacing manner, such people exhibit this protest in their musculature, whose rigidity may imply that "[w]hat they lack, a spontaneous 'No' toward excessive self-sacrifice, is simply expressed physically."[14]

BODY TENSION AND ACUPUNCTURE THERAPY

From an acupuncture-energetic perspective, the increased muscular tonus observed by Alexander is almost always present in all arthritis patients, leading most acupuncturists to focus on creating a smoother muscular functioning and circulation through the muscles in the affected zones. By working directly on this muscular rigidity, acupuncture therapists, like other bodyworkers, gain immediate access to the "psychologic straight jacket" evoked earlier.

As we saw in Chapter 3, Requena's interpretation of acupuncture temperaments implies specific body types that we choose to see as somatic reactional patterns—that is to say, different forms of highly specific "character armors" (Reich). This perspective leads to individualized and specific analysis and treatment of arthritis conditions, including rheumatoid arthritis, all of which figure heavily in the Oriental medical literature.

We see that the major zones affected by acute arthritis are the Yang zones, namely Greater Yang (Small Intestine and Bladder), Lesser Yang (Gallbladder and Triple Heater) and Sunlight Yang (Stomach and Large Intestine), whereas the chronic, truly degenerative types of arthritis that occur systematically and affect every part of the body tend to belong to the Greater Yin (Spleen and Lung) and Lesser Yin (Kidney and Heart) zones.

The Greater Yang reaction pattern reveals muscular rigidity along the Small Intestine and Bladder channels, including the outer aspect of the hand and arm, the scapula and cervical region (where these channels meet), the back of the neck and head, the muscles that run along the spine to the buttocks, and the back of the legs to the outer edge of the foot. These channels cover more somatic territory on the back, and hence dominate, with the Lesser Yang channel, the entire back surface. These zones are precisely those that become rigid when the bodymind feels threatened and is ready to fight back or flee; therefore it is no surprise that these areas are so frequently affected in modern people. The heavy burdens of adulthood, noted by Fetterman, are felt most acutely by persons with imbalances in this Greater Yang zone. They often tend to have problems with will power and authority, adding to the tension in that zone of the body.

A diagnosis of disturbance of the Greater Yang reaction pattern may be made when there is occipital and cervical stiffness or pain, often accompanied by vertical headache, arthritis attacking primarily the cervical and scapula regions and possibly the outside of the hands or feet, and sciatic-like pain or symptoms down the Bladder channel that runs along the back of the legs. Great rigidity of the spine, difficulty bending, frequent stiff neck and shoulders, and reduced neck rotation also are experienced. Owing to the role of the Kidney Organ Function, paired with the Bladder (Foot Greater Yang channel) in maintaining the quality of the bones, the Greater Yang types of arthritis are primarily ankylosing spondylitis, osteoporosis, and osteoarthritis.

When Lesser Yang musculo-skeletal reaction patterns, calling into play the zones energized by the Gallbladder and Triple Heater meridians and Organ functions, lead to arthritis, it will occur along the top of the hand and arm to the shoulder, the trapezius and back of the neck, the mandible and ear and temple regions (Triple Heater Meridian pathway, converging at the temples with the Gallbladder branch), the sides of the head, the rib cage and hip joint, and the outer aspect of the leg and top of the foot (the path of the Gallbladder channel). Arthritis assuming the Lesser Yang reaction pattern will usually attack the shoulder and upper neck or jaws and the hip joint, with chronic spasms in the trapezius and frequent weakness in the hip joint and outer aspect of the legs. Such patients will often report an uneasy, jumpy, contracted sensation along the outer aspect of the leg, beginning at the hip, to the top of the foot to the fourth toe; they may even experience a fractured feeling between the fourth and fifth toes, a few inches above the web (GB 41). Anger or other violent emotional outbursts may lead to an attack along these zones, while repressed rage will tend to weaken this entire zone, predisposing it to later attacks of pain and inflammation. People suffering from this pattern of arthritis often show incredible tightness in the jaws (which are often large and clenched all the time), migraines, and eye pains (especially behind the eyes or in the temples), denoting stiffness all along the zone from the trapezius to the temples that may be accompanied by a real "chip on the shoulder." This type of arthritis will tend to attack the sciatic area as well; people with this pattern often experience difficulty rotating sideways (weakness of the Belt Channel, *Dai Mo*, which is energized by the Gallbladder channel) and will suffer primarily from arthritis of the mandible, shoulders, wrists, and hip. These types of "arthritis" (or *obstruction syndromes* as the Chinese term them) usually are not debilitating, and tend to occur in bouts with quite clear periods in between.

When the Sunlight Yang reaction pattern leads to what would be diagnosed in Western medicine as arthritis, the symptoms will occur along the Large Intestine and Stomach pathways, running along the forearm and front of the shoulder or around the mouth, as well as along the outer aspect of the legs and top of the feet. The most common types of arthritis found when this pattern has been activated are periarthritis of the shoulder joint and gout, according to Requena's research.

Arthritis of a systemic nature, being Yin in nature, will tend to occur in those suffering from weakness in the Greater Yin or Lesser Yin systems (Lung and Spleen and Kidney and Heart, respectively). Both of these functional units are intimately involved in the immune system—that is, with the integrity of the Blood in general and the white blood cells in particular (Greater Yin), and with the genetic endowment (Lesser Yin). Worry, anxiety, and fear, combined with an excessive or depleting lifestyle that does not allow for proper rest and nourishment, tax these two systems directly, thereby weakening the immune system indirectly. Arthritis that occurs in these types of patterns will be degenerative, and will attack all of the joints indiscriminately. Treatment here, unlike that in Yang reaction patterns, must focus on clearing and purifying the Blood, and building Blood and Energy to prevent degeneration. Treatment of these Yin patterns may help significantly in reducing symptoms and even slow down the degenerative process, but will rarely prove truly curative.

In the Yang patterns, on the other hand, acupuncture therapy, if initiated promptly, may totally eliminate the somatic compliance in the affected zone, thereby preventing further arthritic developments.

In my own experience, those suffering from the Yin, chronic sorts of arthritic reaction patterns either are of the sickly type, with clear deficiency of energy from a very young age, or are deficient Spleen or Lung types, who live excessively or are besieged by worries and pressures (especially financial ones) that tax the system, thereby lowering resistence. In the latter type of reaction patterns, true depression is often present, so that the symptoms in the joints may be seen as a kind of depressive reaction, an attempt by the bodymind to ward off stressful agents attacking the body constantly in such a fashion as to make repairs and rebuilding difficult.

The following case demonstrates the benefit of the bodymind-energetic approach in understanding and treating such disorders.

A PHYSICAL STRAIGHT JACKET

A man in his early 40s was referred to me by his physical therapist for a case of recalcitrant temporomandibular joint (TMJ) disease accompanied by severe muscular rigidity throughout the body.

The patient was a school administrator who expressed from the outset the high level of anxiety he experienced at his job, where he was obliged to appear calm and always in control. He had just been assigned to a new school and was meeting with great resistance from other administrators and staff over sweeping changes he had been mandated to implement.

He appeared extremely conscientious about his responsibilities, and voiced concern over the educational welfare of the children if these changes were not effected.

Self-effacing during the interview, he mentioned in a resigned, sad voice that he loved his work "in the service of others," but that his job, like all his previous positions (in social work and in an agency for the elderly), was "incredibly stressful, because you don't know what more people could possibly expect from you!"

The problem in his jaw involved chronic stiffness and pain of the temporomandibular joint, which had been preceded by years of suffering from muscular tightness, spasms in the neck and back of the head, and lower backache. A few times a year his back would still "go out," always under stressful work conditions. He suffered sciatica of the left leg, which in the past had bothered him every few months but had been fine for over a year now. Recently he developed a case of tennis elbow.

The patient was "addicted," in his words, to physical exercise, and he would engage daily in rigorous aerobic exercise and sports. If he missed a day he would grow very agitated and fall into a generally foul temper. He felt that if he didn't exercise frequently, his muscular rigidity would prove incapacitating.

A major issue that came up during the interview was his inability to focus on clear goals concerning his personal life and his inability to make decisions concerning his future. He also stated that he knew his condition would never improve, felt hopeless and resigned to a deteriorating condition, and doubted any therapy would help.

The acupuncture evaluation revealed muscular rigidity along the entire right side of the Small Intestine channel, and the left side of the lower branch of the Bladder channel, bringing into play the entire Greater Yang somatic energetic reaction pattern. Palpation of the pulses revealed a marked deficiency of the Kidney function, with an excess in the Bladder position on the pulse. When asked if he ever suffered pelvic complaints, he responded, visibly embarrassed, that he urinated frequently and would dribble after urinating, had very low sexual capacity verging on impotence, and experienced a generally achy feeling in his kidney area all the time.

Palpation of the abdomen revealed tightness just above the navel, but, more significantly, a hard mass surrounding the navel itself, indicating disturbance in Liver and Kidney energetics, respectively.

The first session focused on the presenting pain and stiffness in the right TMJ zone, with a pattern of points to free up this zone as well as treat the underlying imbalance in Water (Bladder excess/Kidney deficiency) and the Greater Yang reaction pattern as a whole.

The points selected were Small Intestine 19, in the TMJ zone itself, and Small Intestine 18, under the cheekbone, which proved especially sensitive to palpation and is a major focus of Yang reaction patterns affecting the face, as well as additional painful points along the Greater Yang pathway, namely Greater Yang itself, an extra point for the TMJ zone; Bladder 7 on the top of the head; and Bladder 10, in the occipital region on the back of the skull. All were especially sensitive to pressure and well suited for this sort of muscular rigidity. Distal points, to consolidate the effect of the treatment in freeing the TMJ zone while supporting underlying imbalances, were Small Intestine 3 and Bladder 62, a Greater Yang combination bringing into play the Yang extra vessels of the Governing Vessel and the Yang Heel Channel, especially effective in musculoskeletal reaction patterns of this type; and Kidney 3 and 7, the source and tonification points of the Kidney channel respectively, to build Kidney energy.

When the patient returned for his second treatment a week later, he stated that he was much worse, and had had a frontal headache the night after the treatment, a problem that used to plague him years before. He reported that the second day after treatment the pain in his lower back and sciatica, which had been absent for a long time, returned especially on the left side, and he had a gnawing, achy sensation in his lower left groin area. Understandably, he expressed great reluctance to continue acupuncture therapy, given this return or exacerbation of old complaints, until I reminded him of what I had explained as he left after the first treatment—that often old symptoms do return, or current ones grow temporarily worse, as the bodymind is prodded to remember these old maladaptive patterns and works to return to a more appropriate functional state. I assured him that such an aggravation of symptoms would be very short-lived and that I would select a pattern of points for this second treatment that was unlikely to lead to such dramatic flare-ups. It would focus on restoring balance in the Water phase, to allow energy to move from the overactive, congested Bladder (surface) zone to the deeper, weak Kidney function. Treatment consisted of Bladder 58 and Kidney 3, a pattern of treatment to move energy from the Bladder to the Kidney channel known as internal/external regulation, and Bladder 23 and 28, associated points for the Bladder and Kidney functions themselves. I asked him to close his eyes and imagine that his surface, all along the affected zones (which I traced on him to give him a recollection of the exact pathways involved) was teeming with energy, and that as he breathed more and more calmly during the treatment this excessive activity would calm down, and with it, his muscular rigidity would dissolve as the excess of energy now flowed to the deeper Kidney pathway and down to the pelvic zone to clear out any obstructions there.

On his third visit, two weeks later, he reported with definite optimism that the jaw remained better. He had not suffered so dramatically after this treatment and had felt a general lessening of muscular tension throughout his body. His sciatica was almost totally gone, his back felt stronger, and he felt much more focused and less anxious in general. The only negative sign was that the pelvic achiness was worse.

He was anxious about this; I referred him to his internist to check for prostatitis or some other condition that would explain these symptoms, and the results of the medical examination proved negative. Nevertheless, the physician suspected a non-specific prostatitis, and suggested a trial of antibiotic therapy in a few weeks if the symptoms did not clear up. It should be noted that when such symptoms grow worse and remain worse after the administration of acupuncture therapy, it is often due to an actual organic obstruction or infection, which must be cleared up in order for the acupuncture to be effective.

The third treatment focused on freeing up the congested pelvic zone, while still treating the underlying Kidney/Bladder disharmony and Kidney deficiency as well as the entire Greater Yang reaction pattern. The pattern of points selected consisted of Kidney 11, the precise area of his pelvic pain, just above the pubic bone slightly off the midline; Kidney 16, just lateral to the navel on both sides to free up the tightness in the umbilical region; Conception Vessel 3, 4, and 6, points along the midline associated with Greater Yang (Small Intestine and Bladder Alarm points) and Kidney functions, along with the distal points Bladder 64 and Kidney 3, source points for the Water functions; and Heart 7, linked with the Fire function and the Small Intestine pathway.

On the fourth visit, two weeks later, his complaints had virtually disappeared and he was extremely hopeful about his condition. The pelvic pain had gone by the day after treatment, and his muscular rigidity had lessened even further. He also reported that he felt less driven to do daily exercise, which he realized was a way of maintaining focus on his external muscular system rather than on deeper body-mind issues. These concerns, which he had not voiced previously, included a fear that if he did not change his line of work and get out of the service professions, he was going to develop a serious illness; incredible anger, difficult to contain, at the staff of the school for resisting his efforts to improve the programs for the children; great sadness over the lack of a meaningful love relationship, which he realized he needed badly; and an overriding fear, which he had repressed much of his adult life, that he would die of cancer of the prostate as his father had.

I scheduled him for four treatments over the next year, one at every change of season, to follow up on the excellent results of the acupuncture therapy. I referred him to a psychologist who utilizes relaxation techniques, hypnotherapy, visualization, and short-term counseling for psychosomatic conditions. This would enable him to work on the emotional issues brought up during acupuncture therapy, and learn self-help techniques to gain a sense of control over his body—especially his pelvic zone, which was now filled with fear of cancer.

A year later his TMJ and other musculoskeletal complaints had not returned, except on two brief occasions when he was able to control the problem himself. In addition, he had just become engaged to be married.

TREATMENT FROM THE SOMATIC SIDE

In the case of musculoskeletal reaction patterns, which often bring into play very precise somatic-energetic mechanisms (a muscle spasm, inflammation, swelling in a particular area, or a general increase in muscle tonus), the best approach seems to be from the somatic-energetic, rather than the psychoenergetic, side. While psychotherapists may well help such individuals to deal with core personality and behavioral issues, or to get in touch with their unconscious drives and motivations—and may even, with the help of bio-feedback or other relaxation techniques, bring about relief in the musculoskeletal symptoms themselves—the psychological approach cannot hone in on the precise somatic zones affected. These must often be treated locally.

Whereas a psychotherapist may spend months getting to the psychological root of a patient's suffering from arthritis of the hip and jaw, for example, an acupuncture therapist can ascertain in one or two sessions whether the zone affected is part of the Greater Yang or Lesser Yang reaction pattern, and then treat this zone with precision. Such treatment will be highly individualized, and is often of rapid and decisive help, especially in the Yang reaction patterns.

Those who treat from the side of the psyche would do well to refer their patients with chronic pain and arthritis for acupuncture or other somatic-energetic therapies. The relief gained in somatic-energetic release of the bodymind obstructions will free up energy for the psychological work; in certain cases, such somatic release may even lead to decisive psychological insights with release occurring spontaneously on that level as well.

It is with this sort of somatic-energetic integrative work in mind that Stanley Keleman, a pioneer of somatic psychology and director of the Center for Energetic Studies in Berkeley, California, speaks of "emotional anatomy."[15]

In his view, the body process embodies the emotional life of the individual and is concerned with "patterns of good feeling, patterns of stress and distress, and patterns of emotion . . . organized as particular kinds of pulsation . . . . Motility has to be appreciated from the inside; it is the vitality of the pulsatory pattern, the power and intensity of organ pulsations that give energy and personal identity . . . . Feeling and sensation that arise from the inside tell us 'this is who I am.' Self-image is based upon patterns of sensation from the interior."[16]

In this somatic rendition of the concept of body-image, we see again the concept of bodily felt sense, first articulated by Gendlin, a phenomenological psychologist. From infancy, in this view, "We know ourselves from the inside out . . . . Internal metabolism is a way of thinking. *A way of thinking precedes words* . . ."[17]

In the bodymind-energetic approach, we emphasize the bodily felt sense, which acupuncture energetic therapy is especially capable of evoking, as the source from which the therapeutic change will arise. There are those who believe that in needling certain acupuncture pathways, known as the Eight Extraordinary Vessels, we enable a person to connect with prenatal patterns of being. In acupuncture embryological theory, these eight pathways develop out of the undifferentiated egg, constituting the first lines of force and channels for the free flow of cosmic and bodily energies.[18] In a similar vein, Keleman portrays early embryological development, in which "all tissues and organs are intimately connected; the heart and the brain are just two surfaces apart. The heartbeat is tattooed right on the brain. No nerves are necessary. As development continues there are *vestiges of remembered contact*. This is information, an intimate knowing."[19]

It is precisely this sort of intimate knowledge that acupuncture-energetic therapy, practiced from a bodymind-integrative perspective, enables a patient to achieve—knowledge that belonged to the patient all along. From the bodymind-energetic perspective, then, we never focus on treating diseases but rather seek to guide our patients to relearn what they already know, to remember vestiges of a being-at-one-with-the-world, to obtain a recollection of being that is stored deep within their bodies.

The ultimate question that serves as a point of departure for such a therapeutic process, a question initially raised by Nietzsche and taken up again by phenomenologists such as Heidegger and Merleau-Ponty, is whether the treatment of human suffering is finally capable of existing as a process of *being-with* those who come for therapy (help), rather than as a process that reduces this encounter with a person's suffering to a mere treatment of disease. Many medical practitioners are beginning to raise this question, which perhaps means that a philosophy of health and well-being is emerging to replace a deadening science of pathology and disease. In such a philosophy, medical therapy would begin with the establishment of a new paradigm of health care that includes re-education of the general public, starting with education of our children, concerning the relationship between mind and body. This education would emerge from a fundamental critique of the Cartesian dualism between mind and body, subject and object, and would postulate a primary unity among these realms. While medical and mental health practitioners would doubtless still specialize, more on the side of the soma or more on the side of the psyche, respectively, they would all be cognizant of this underlying philosophy of bodymind unity, and true collaboration would exist among them in order to design treatment plans with their clients capable of achieving bodymind integration in each case.

The question these practitioners would ask themselves and their patients would simply be whether "[we] can locate within our adult bodies a *felt sense* of that original wholeness, that matrix of eternity" harkening back to the as yet undifferentiated body image of the infant, "as large and undelimited as the cosmos."[20]

NOTES

1. Alexander and French, *Studies in Psychosomatic Medicine*, p. 496.
2. Ibid., p. 496.

3. Ibid., Leon J. Saul, "A Clinical Note on a Mechanism of Psychogenic Back Pain," pp. 544–545.
4. Ibid., p. 545.
5. Pelletier, *Mind as Healer, Mind as Slayer*, p. 150.
6. Ibid.
7. French and Alexander, *Studies in Psychosomatic Medicine*, pp. 489–498.
8. Ibid., p. 490.
9. Ibid., p. 490.
10. Ibid.
11. Ibid., p. 492.
12. Ibid., p. 494.
13. Ziegler, *Archetypal Medicine*, p. 112.
14. Ibid., p. 114.
15. Cf. Stanley Keleman, *Emotional Anatomy: The Structure of Experience*. Berkeley, California, Center Press, 1985.
16. Ibid., p. 28.
17. Ibid.
18. Cf. Claude Larre, Jean Schatz and Elizabeth Rochat de la Vallee, *Survey of Traditional Chinese Medicine*, translated from the French by Sarah Stang. Paris, Institut Ricci, 1986, pp. 142–146.
19. *Emotional Anatomy*, p. 12.
20. David Michael Levin, quoting Neumann, *The Body's Recollection of Being*, pp. 219–220. Cf. also p. 235, "On the education of our children in bodily felt awareness."

11

Bodymind Transformations

The human being, not the patient, goes to the doctor, the
human being, not the patient, asks for help.[1]
Georg Groddeck

In developing the foregoing phenomenology of bodymind energetics,
a relationship between acupuncture-somatic energetics and psychosomatic psychoenergetics was established, and the implications of this
combined approach for therapists of the psyche and therapists of the
soma should be apparent.

Psychotherapists and counselors, who often possess exquisite skills
of listening and hearing, will be enabled by the bodymind-energetic
perspective to adopt another viewpoint aimed at palpating and feeling the repercussions and sources of psychic transformations in the
bodies of their clients, grounding their analyses more solidly in the
soma.

Bodyworkers, including acupuncture therapists who perceive
acupuncture solely as a physical therapy, will find that such an approach will underscore the crucial role of psychic energies as they come
to bear on bodily functions and emphasize the intimate relation between therapies of the body and therapies of the mind. They will learn
to listen with a third ear, rendering their touch more probing and their
treatment more profound.

For some psychiatrists and psychiatric clinicians, it is hoped that
such an approach will kindle a desire to become ever more philosophical as they hone their clinical skills.

Physicians interested in holistic health—ultimately including all medical doctors of every speciality—may see in this perspective new avenues of thought about energetic modes of therapy and new roles for the physician of the future in collaborating with all therapists who work to foster the psychosomatic unity of the patient.

Lay readers, finally, may be confirmed by such an approach in their own often subtle *recognitions* of the psychosomatic complex in their own symptoms and ailments, and led to develop thoughts of their own about the nature of health and their own role in maintaining health and well-being.

The bodymind-energetic approach encourages the clinician, with sharply attuned senses of feeling, hearing and seeing, to allow those resonances to occur that open to the complex being of the person who seeks help, and to realize that "at the first touch the patient's thoughts and attention are diverted into other channels . . . . Thus he gradually begins to realize that in a diagnosis, e.g., in the term 'heart disease,' there is included a number of different things which are more important for treatment and recovery than the anatomical condition, that the sick man, his functional capacity, and his return to a useful career are the real objects of medical treatment, that his state is more important than the name of his disease, and that in disease we are dealing with a changing situation, since illness is an organic process of life, not a thing that is fixed and dead."[2]

Such a perspective situates specific complaints or diseases on the psychosomatic-energetic continuum, ranging from essentially somatic-energetic conditions, where a somatic therapy may provide a more useful starting point, to psychoenergetic conditions more readily accessible from the side of the psyche. The point of this approach is that regardless of the starting place for therapy, both ways in must often be combined, in order to reach the core of the psychosomatic complex.

TRACING ENERGY TRANSFORMATIONS

A full fifty years ago, Dr. Flanders Dunbar, in her monumental *Emotions and Bodily Changes*, concluded with the suggestion to her physician colleagues that the basic components of the psychotherapeutic approach—suggestion, re-education, and catharsis—bespoke the need for including the psychosomatic perspective within the general field of medicine and the training of physicians. Referring back thirty years to the groundbreaking work of Groddeck in this domain, Dunbar stressed that "a topic of fundamental importance is that of the *psychic component in, and correct use of, massage, exercise, physiotherapy, baneother-*

apy, and drug therapy in general."[3] Unfortunately these techniques were becoming very mechanistic, and we now see that the full potential for these somatic techniques, except for the use of drugs, has been almost totally ignored by modern psychiatry. The psychodynamic spirit inherent in the "wild army" of physicians and psychiatrists from Groddeck and Deutsch to Dunbar and Alexander was fast replaced, in American psychiatry, by the new psychiatric medications. Few psychiatrists, clinical psychologists, or psychiatric clinicians today read Groddeck, Dunbar, or Alexander. This ignorance of the early psychosomatic work appears to have increased in direct proportion to the rise in popularity of psychiatric medications, which subdued certain mental illnesses and emptied the asylums of certain groups of patients and are now called into play freely to treat the anxieties of everyday life as readily as the far rarer psychoses.

Excited by the use of Xanax in the "management" of panic attacks, a psychiatric resident will rarely ponder the existential nature of this panic or the precise ways in which this panic manifests in the body of a tortured soul. In "managing" the panic, a psychiatrist of pharmacological persuasion has little time for the psychosomatic complexities involved in even the smallest anxiety.

Drugs, it would appear, have all but replaced human touch in psychiatry as well as in general medicine. How many psychiatrists, internists, or specialists employ touching somatic therapy to complement their drug therapy? It is ironic that in this age of highly technological medicine, drug therapy rather than therapies of touch has become the "soft" therapy. The often unforeseeable effects of bio-chemical intervention, operating within a complex body with a mind of its own, often work regardless of the physician's good intentions to produce serious side effects or even a totally new condition requiring additional medical intervention (iatrogenesis). With no "softer," more human therapies available, modern medicine takes on an air of daring that only enhances its claim to being radically scientific and true.

The current practice of psychiatry belies the vision held by Dunbar. She thought it logical that the therapies of the soma would be incorporated with those of the psyche, emphasizing only "that each be employed consciously, not for itself but as part of a general therapeutic scheme based on accurate (psychosomatic) diagnosis of the situation at hand."[4]

In the 1930s, hypnosis in particular, and *suggestion* in general, were considered to be "both dishonest and unscientific, being discussed usually in connection with cults."[5] And yet suggestion is always utilized, consciously or unconsciously, by any therapist or physician treating a patient. Consider the suggestion involved in telling a patient suffering from low back syndrome due to compressed vertebrae that "if the muscle relaxants and pain killers and traction do not help, surgery will be the only option."

This sort of *threat suggestion* is utilized frequently, albeit probably unwittingly, by many surgeons. It is fortunate that some are coming to realize the futile nature of back surgery in such cases and are sending their patients to chiropractors, acupuncture therapists, bio-feedback technicians, or psychotherapists, to get at the complex physical and psychological issues at the core of a back that cannot stand up under the pressures of life.

What burdens there must be placed upon this back, the bodymind-energetic approach would maintain, to render a person immobile (and hence physically incapable of carrying out life's tasks)! It is a frequent occurrence in any acupuncturist's practice to be confronted with back sufferers only a few months after surgery for removal of the compressed vertebra, as if the pressures of life cease to bother the person once pressure on a vertebra has been removed! A surgeon who saw the spine as the backbone of the personality and the support for the spirit, not just as the structure holding up the physical organism, might be wary of cutting into it without exploring the full range of psychosomatic issues involved. For only when the backbending burdens have been acknowledged, in my experience, will blood and energy circulate freely, thereby supporting the psyche and the body properly.

Some surgeons may scorn the idea of using suggestion, or of helping the patient reflect on the burdens that are depriving him of "backbone" and character; they may criticize such an approach as a mere placebo that denies the patient proper medical management of the pain, as if placebo were not an almost magical self-healing power unleashed, in a therapeutic situation, in the patient's own bodymind, owing to the conscious use of empathy and the personality of the physician or therapist.

As analytically inspired psychiatrists like Dunbar early realized, "of equal therapeutic importance to a consideration of the organism as a whole, and the organism–environment relation, is the *inclusion by the physician of his own personality* and behavior in the catalogue of his therapeutic armamentarium."[6] Technical control of the personality factor is indeed the aim of psychotherapy. By controlling transference and countertransference, the intention is to make use of the personality of the therapist in the patient–therapist relation. This is not an issue for psychotherapy alone, Dunbar maintains, as "this factor enters into every therapeutic activity of the physician; and if he is to handle it in the interests of his therapeutic program he must add to his study of medicine and of people a thoroughgoing knowledge of himself."[7]

In all fairness, medical knowledge at present is more complex than that dealt with fifty years ago, so that while it may be impossible for all physicians to undertake such studies, along with grueling medical and scientific studies, they could be exposed to these issues and taught when and how to refer to other therapists of psyche and soma more appropriately situated to deal with these issues. Such a collaboration, which we believe to be the model for the future of the new bodymind paradigm of health maintenance we have been discussing, will include an inquiry into the meaning of the patient's symptom or complaint.

"Grossly," Dunbar states, this meaning "is to be understood in terms of the relationship to the environment and the *total energy economy*. Disease is in itself a language which if understood makes it possible to trace *energy transformations* taking place within the organism, awareness and understanding of which may be of vital significance for the patient's ultimate health."[8]

DYNAMIC VISION

Because of the absence of any adequate somatic-energetic therapeutic model, as we showed in Chapter 4, this psychodynamic vision has lost much of its force over the past seventy-five years in the treatment of psychosomatic disorders.

We believe that this loss is due in no small part to the fact that these psychosomatic issues have remained within a very restricted medical community. Freud and Jung were distressed by the over-medicalization of psychoanalysis and psychotherapy, and feared that philosophy and poetry might be lost in the process. Fortunately, we believe, psychotherapy, because of an immense popular need and desire, has expanded far beyond the confines of the psychiatric medical community. But in this expansion, the hard philosophical and existential issues reviewed in Chapter 4 and here have been all but lost to a decidedly watered-down humanistic perspective. The bodymind-energetic approach restores the right to philosophical inquiry for psychiatric nurses, social workers, and lay therapists, and (we hope) makes up in some small way for a rather strong anti-intellectual climate in the psychotherapeutic realm.

To their credit, non-physician psychotherapists have tended to be far more open to bodywork and energetics, realizing the role of a combined treatment plan aimed at treating the soma as well. Just as the soma can be treated from the psychic side, these therapists realize that we can also speak "of the *treatment of the psyche from the somatic side*."[9] Therapists sharing the bodymind-energetic vision "recognize the unity of psyche and soma. If this concept is correct, it is obvious that every disease can be understood and treated not only psychically, but also somatically."[10] "There is no such thing," Dunbar states, "as a purely psychic illness or a purely physical one, but only a *living event* taking place in a living organism which is itself alive only by virtue of the fact that in it psychic and somatic are united in a unity."[11]

The bodymind-energetic approach was evident throughout Dunbar's work. Ultimately she felt that "every physician [and therapist] should have some working knowledge of such concepts as that of the mind as an environmental inclusion (invasion of culture), the significance of the body image, and the mechanisms, psychological as well as physiological, by means of which energy transformations take place."[12]

These are prophetic words, but unfortunately they have fallen mainly on deaf ears over the past two decades. Dunbar's and Groddeck's books discussed here can only be found on the shelves of a few rare book shops, and even Alexander's work is hard to find. The bodymind-energetic approach is therefore a tribute, on one level, to this work, and we shall consider this book to have been successful if it moves some clinicians to explore the issues raised in this rich literature.

*   *   *

I have come full circle in my own exploration of the psychosomatic question, from my particular position as an acupuncture therapist trained in philosophy and fascinated by this psychosomatic literature even before my study of acupuncture.

Early in my study of acupuncture I became weary of the Oriental medical discussion of the psyche, and returned to the Western psychosomatic literature to ponder the question of the relationship between mind and body from my own Western perspective.

In my training and in my beginning practice I remained very faithful to the somatic-energetic nature of acupuncture therapy; initially I saw this modality of treatment as a superb form of physical therapy. This stance was also taken out of wariness toward my underlying fascination with the psychic side of illness. That is, I realized the need to resist an overly psychological approach so that I might hone new physical skills and learn to perceive energetic dynamics with precision.

The acupuncture training institute[13] that I founded and currently direct started from this somatic-energetic perspective, which still lies at the core of its curriculum. Over the past five years the institute has served as a forum in which larger issues, concerning acupuncture as a bodymind-integrative mode of therapy, have been addressed. In a restricted sense, then, this book is directed to my students and faculty, and to American acupuncturists more generally—to excite them to explore this fascinating clinical literature and to come to grips, from their own positions, with the bodymind question as it affects the practice of acupuncture therapy in the West. Doubtless some schools will wish to train somatic-energetic acupuncturists, while others will seek to train psychoenergetic therapists of this ancient healing art. It is my hope that those of both persuasions will work together to forge a properly behavioral, bodymind-integrative acupuncture therapy tailored to the unique needs of Western clients.

This book represents my own attempt to develop an approach to acupuncture therapy consistent with my particular position on the bodymind continuum, and is thus a personal venture aimed at stimulating others to set out on *the way*.

Those who wish to combine energetic therapies of the East with a Western appreciation of things psychological are obliged to confront the psychosomatic question in terms that are true to their own Western heritage. In this sense, the philosophical inquiries of those Western thinkers cited in this book are clearly as relevant as the philosophical concepts underlying traditional Oriental medicine, if not more so. Ultimately and unavoidably, we Western practitioners of acupuncture therapy will forge a practice true to our own Western body and spirit.

On a broader scale, I hope that some readers may be moved to explore different methods by which therapies of the psyche and the body process can be integrated in novel ways, thereby contributing to the establishment of a new paradigm of bodymind-integrative therapy infused with a feeling for energetics.

One thing is certain. In adopting a bodymind-energetic perspective, practitioners of every persuasion and clinical orientation will realize that their work occupies a privileged, human domain. Here the recurrent meeting of the souls of therapist and client energizes both and culminates in great respect for the limitless capacities of the bodymind for health and healing.

NOTES

1. Groddeck, *The Meaning of Illness*, p. 244.
2. Ibid., p. 237.
3. Dunbar, p. 417.
4. Ibid., pp. 417–418.
5. Ibid., p. 418.
6. Ibid., p. 419.
7. Ibid.
8. Ibid., pp. 422–423 (emphasis ours).
9. Ibid., p. 425, referring to comments of Heyer.
10. Ibid., p. 426.
11. Ibid., p. 428.
12. Ibid., footnote 17, p. 423.
13. The Tri-State Institute of Traditional Chinese Acupuncture in Stamford, Connecticut.

Epilogue

Thinking itself is a way. We respond to the way only by remaining underway. To be underway on the way in order to clear the way — that is one thing. The other thing is to take a position somewhere along the road, and there make conversation about whether, and how, earlier and later stretches of the way may be different, and in their difference might even be incompatible — incompatible, that is, for those who never walk the way, nor ever set out on it, but merely take up a position outside it, there forever to formulate ideas and make talk about the way. . . . In order to get underway, we do have to set out. This is meant in a double sense: for one thing, we have to open ourselves to the emerging prospect and direction of the way itself; and then, we must get on the way, that is, must take the steps by which alone the way becomes a way.

M. Heidegger, *What Is Called Thinking*.
New York, Harper & Row, 1968,
pp. 168–169.

Selected Bibliography

Alexander, Franz, *Psychosomatic Medicine: Its Principles and Applications*. New York, W. W. Norton, 1950.

Alexander, Franz, *Fundamentals of Psychoanalysis*. New York, W. W. Norton, 1963.

Alexander, F., and French, T. M., *Studies in Psychosomatic Medicine: An Approach to the Causes and Treatment of Vegetative Disturbances*. New York, Ronald Press, 1948.

Ammon, Günter, *Psychoanalysis and Psychosomatics* (translated by Susan Hecker Ray). New York, Springer Publishing Co., 1979.

Becker, Robert, *The Body Electric*. New York, William Morrow & Co., 1985.

Boss, Medard, *Existential Foundations of Medicine and Psychology* (translated from the German by Stephen Conway and Anne Cleaves). New York, Jason Aronson, 1979.

Cannon, W. E., *The Wisdom of the Body*. New York, W. W. Norton, 1932.

Capra, Fritjof, *The Turning Point: Science, Society and the Rising Culture*. New York, Bantam Books, 1982.

Chamfrault, A., and Nguyen Van Nghi, *L'energétique humaine en médecine Chinoise*. Angouleme, Imprimerie de la Charente, 1975.

Cole, K. C., *Sympathetic Vibrations*. New York, Bantam Books, 1985.

Connelly, Dianne M., *Traditional Acupuncture: The Law of the Five Elements*. Columbia, Maryland, Center for Traditional Acupuncture, 1979.

Cousins, Norman, *Anatomy of an Illness*. New York, Bantam Books, 1981.

Deleuze, Gilles, and Guattari, Felix, *Anti-Oedipus: Capitalism and Schizophrenia* (translated from the French by Robert Hurley, Helen R. Lane, and Mark Seem with a preface by Michel Foucault and an introduction by Mark Seem). Minneapolis, University of Minnesota Press, 1983.

De Morant, George Soulie, *L'Acupuncture Chinoise*. Paris, Maloine, 1937.

Dossey, Larry, *Space, Time and Medicine*. Boulder, Colorado, Shambala, 1982.

Dossey, Larry, *Beyond Illness*. Boulder, Colorado, Shambala, 1984.

Dunbar, H. Flanders, *Emotions and Bodily Changes: A Survey on Literature of Psychosomatic Interrelationships, 1910–1933*. New York, Columbia University Press, 1935.

Epstein, Gerald, *Waking Dream Therapy*. New York, Human Sciences Press, 1984.

Fulder, Stephen, *The Tao of Medicine*. New York, Destiny Books, 1980.

Frank, Jerome D., *Persuasion and Healing*. New York, Schocken Books, 1974.

Groddeck, Georg, *The Meaning of Illness: Selected Analytic Writings* (translated from the German by Gertrud Mander). New York, International Universities Press, 1977.

Groddeck, Georg, *The Book of the It* (translated by V. M. E. Collins). New York, Vintage, 1965.

Grossman, Richard, *The Other Medicines*. New York, Doubleday, 1985.

Heidegger, Martin, *What is Called Thinking?* New York, Harper & Row, 1968.

Illich, Ivan, *Medical Nemesis: The Expropriation of Health*. New York, Pantheon, 1976.

Kaptchuk, Ted J., *The Web That Has No Weaver: Understanding Chinese Medicine*. New York, Congdon & Weed, 1982.

Keleman, Stanley, *Emotional Anatomy*. Berkeley, California, Center Press, 1985.

Larre, C., Schatz, J., and Rochat de la Vallee, E., *Survey of Traditional Chinese Medicine* (translated from the French by Sarah Elizabeth Stang). Traditional Acupuncture Foundation, Columbia, Maryland, and Institut Ricci, Paris, 1986.

Low, Royston, *The Secondary Vessels of Acupuncture: A Detailed Account of Their Energies, Meridians and Control Points*. New York, Thorsons Publishers, 1983.

Mann, Felix, *Acupuncture: The Ancient Chinese Art of Healing and How it Works Scientifically*. New York, Random House, 1973.

Nietzsche, Friedrich, *On the Genealogy of Morals* (translated from the German by Walter Kaufmann). New York, Vintage Books, 1969.

Nietzsche, Friedrich, *Beyond Good and Evil* (translated from the German by Walter Kaufmann). New York, Vintage Books, 1966.

Pelletier, Kenneth R., *Mind as Healer, Mind as Slayer: A Holistic Approach to Preventing Stress Disorders*. New York, Delta Books, 1977.

Porkert, Manfred, *The Theoretical Foundations of Chinese Medicine*. Cambridge, Massachusetts, M. I. T. Press, 1974.

Requena, Yves, *Terrains et Pathologie en Médecine Chinoise*, Volumes 1 (1980) and 2 (1982). Parish, Maloine. Volume 1 has been published in English by Paradigm Publications, Brookline, Massachusetts as *Terrains and Pathology in Acupuncture*, 1986.

Sacks, Oliver, *The Man Who Mistook His Wife for a Hat*. New York, E. P. Dutton, 1985.

Selye, H., *The Stress of Life*. New York, McGraw-Hill, 1956.

Starr, Paul, *The Social Transformation of American Medicine*. New York, Harper & Row, 1982.

Weil, Andrew, *Health and Healing: Understanding Conventional and Alternative Medicine*. Boston, Houghton Mifflin Co., 1983.

Winnicott, D. W., *The Maturational Processes and the Facilitating Environment*. London, Hogarth Press, 1965.

Seem, Mark D., *Acupuncture Energetics: A Workbook for Diagnostics and Treatment*. New York, Thorsons Publishers, 1987.

Seem, Mark D., *The Logic of Power: An Essay on the Work of M. Foucault, G. Deleuze, and F. Guattari*. Doctoral Dissertation, State University of New York at Buffalo, 1976 (University Microfilms).

Yuasa, Yasuo, *The Body: Toward an Eastern Mind-Body Theory* (translated from the Japanese by Nagatomo Shigenori and Thomas Kasulis). Albany, New York, State University of New York Press, 1987.

Ziegler, Alfred J., *Archetypal Medicine* (translated from the German by Gary V. Hartman). Dallas, Texas, Spring Publications, 1983.

MARK D. SEEM received his doctorate in French Studies from the State University of New York at Buffalo, where he studied with Michel Foucault and wrote a dissertation on the Nietzschean concepts of power and force in modern French philosophy. Dr. Seem is the co-translator of, and wrote the introduction to, Deleuze and Guattari's *Anti-Oedipus: Capitalism & Schizophrenia*, during the translation of which he trained for a short while at the innovative La Borde clinic in France. Subsequent to finishing his dissertation, he worked with the mentally ill and retarded, taught psychology, and trained mental hygiene therapy aides in a state institution, while beginning his formal study of acupuncture. Dr. Seem trained at and graduated from the Quebec Institute of Acupuncture, during which time he worked as an acupuncture assistant in two clinics in New York. Dr. Seem is the founder and President of the Tri-State Institute of Traditional Chinese Acupuncture in Stamford, Connecticut, an institute for the training of acupuncture therapists, and is a frequent lecturer at other acupuncture institutes and conferences. Dr. Seem is past-president of the National Council of Acupuncture Schools and Colleges and a commissioner on the National Commission for the Certification of Acupuncturists, from which he is a Board Certified Diplomate in Acupuncture. He has written several articles on acupuncture education and is the author of *Acupuncture Energetics: A Workbook for Diagnostics and Treatment* (Thorsons, 1987). Dr. Seem has a bodymind acupuncture-energetic practice in New York City.

JOAN KAPLAN received her Master's Degree in Psychology from the New School for Social Research, where she also completed a clinical externship. Ms. Kaplan has worked as a counselor in a women's health center, trained as a lay midwife, and worked in the Special Services division of a college for non-traditional students in New York City. Currently she is focusing on her writing activities as well as caring for her two children.

Mark Seem and Joan Kaplan live with their two children, Illyan and Anya Kaplan-Seem, in New York City.

INDEX